T0226714

Sleep And Driving

Editor

WALTER T. McNICHOLAS

SLEEP MEDICINE CLINICS

www.sleep.theclinics.com

Consulting Editor
TEOFILO LEE-CHIONG Jr

December 2019 • Volume 14 • Number 4

ELSEVIER

1600 John F. Kennedy Boulevard • Suite 1800 • Philadelphia, Pennsylvania, 19103-2899

http://www.theclinics.com

SLEEP MEDICINE CLINICS Volume 14, Number 4
December 2019, ISSN 1556-407X, ISBN-13: 978-0-323-70880-7

Editor: Colleen Dietzler
Developmental Editor: Donald Mumford

Sleep Medicine Clinics (ISSN 1556-407X) is published quarterly by Elsevier Inc., 360 Park Avenue South, New York, NY 10010-1710. Months of issue are March, June, September and December. Business and Editorial Offices: 1600 John F. Kennedy Blvd., Ste. 1800, Philadelphia, PA 19103-2899. Customer Service Office: 3251 Riverport Lane, Maryland Heights, MO 63043. Periodicals postage paid at New York, NY and additional mailing offices. Subscription prices are $212.00 per year (US individuals), $100.00 (US students), $486.00 (US institutions), $264.00 (Canadian individuals), $252.00 (international individuals) $135.00 (Canadian and international students), $551.00 (Canadian institutions) and $551.00 (International institutions). Foreign air speed delivery is included in all *Clinics* subscription prices. All prices are subject to change without notice. **POSTMASTER:** Send change of address to *Sleep Medicine Clinics*, Elsevier Health Sciences Division, Subscription Customer Service, 3251 Riverport Lane, Maryland Heights, MO 63043. Customer Service: **Tel: 1-800-654-2452 (U.S. and Canada); 314-447-8871 (outside U.S. and Canada). Fax: 314-447-8029. E-mail: journalscustomerservice-usa@elsevier.com (for print support); journalsonlinesupport-usa@elsevier.com (for online support).**

Reprints. For copies of 100 or more of articles in this publication, please contact the Commercial Reprints Department, Elsevier Inc., 360 Park Avenue South, New York, NY 10010-1710. Tel.: 212-633-3874; Fax: 212-633-3820; E-mail: reprints@elsevier.com.

Sleep Medicine Clinics is covered in *MEDLINE/PubMed (Index Medicus)*.

SLEEP MEDICINE CLINICS

SERIES OF RELATED INTEREST

Clinics in Chest Medicine
Available at: https://www.chestmed.theclinics.com/

THE CLINICS ARE AVAILABLE ONLINE!
Access your subscription at:
www.theclinics.com

Contributors

CONSULTING EDITOR

TEOFILO LEE-CHIONG Jr, MD
Professor of Medicine, National Jewish Health,
University of Colorado Denver, Denver,
Colorado, USA; Chief Medical Liaison, Philips
Respironics, Pennsylvania, USA

EDITOR

WALTER T. McNICHOLAS, MD
Newman Professor, School of Medicine,
University College Dublin, Department of
Respiratory and Sleep Medicine, St. Vincent's
Hospital Group, Dublin, Ireland; First Affiliated
Hospital of Guangzhou Medical University,
Guangzhou, China

AUTHORS

TORBJÖRN ÅKERSTEDT, PhD
Senior Professor, Department of Clinical
Neuroscience, Karolinska Institute, Stress
Research Institute, Stockholm University,
Stockholm, Sweden

MARIA R. BONSIGNORE, MD, FERS
Associate Professor of Respiratory Medicine,
Respiratory Division, Dipartimento di
Promozione Della Salute, Materno-Infantile,
Medicina Interna e Specialistica di Eccellenza
"G. D'Alessandro" (PROMISE), University of
Palermo, Istituto per la Ricerca e l'innovazione
Biomedica (IRIB), National Research Council
(CNR) Palermo, Italy

GABRIELA CAETANO, MD
Assistance Publique Hôpitaux de Paris, APHP-
5, Hôtel-Dieu de Paris, Centre du Sommeil et
de la Vigilance, Paris, France

JENNIFER M. CORI, BA(Hons), PhD
Post-doctoral Fellow, Institute for Breathing
and Sleep, Austin Health, Heidelberg, Victoria,
Australia

**AKSHAY DWARAKANATH, MD, MRCP
(Respiratory Medicine), FRCP (Edin)**
Consultant Respiratory Physician, Department
of Respiratory Medicine, Sleep and Non-
invasive Ventilation Service, Mid Yorkshire
Hospitals NHS Trust, Wakefield, West
Yorkshire, United Kingdom

MARK W. ELLIOTT, MD, FERS
Consultant Respiratory Physician, Department
of Respiratory Medicine, Sleep and Non-
invasive Ventilation Service, St. James's
University Hospital, Leeds, West Yorkshire,
United Kingdom

FRANCESCO FANFULLA, MD
Respiratory Function and Sleep Medicine Unit,
Istituti Clinici Scientifici Maugeri IRCCS, Pavia,
Italy

INGO FIETZE, Dr med
Professor, Medical Director, Sleep Medicine
Center, Charité – Universitätsmedizin Berlin,
Berlin, Germany

INDIRA GURUBHAGAVATULA, MD, MPH
Associate Professor, Division of Sleep
Medicine, Perelman School of Medicine,
University of Pennsylvania, Sleep Section,
Crescenz VA Medical Center, Philadelphia,
Pennsylvania, USA

WILLIAM J. HORREY, PhD
Group Leader, Traffic Research Group, AAA
Foundation for Traffic Safety, Washington, DC,
USA

MARK E. HOWARD, MBBS, PhD
Director, Institute for Breathing and Sleep,
Austin Health, Heidelberg, Victoria, Australia;
University of Melbourne, Parkville, Victoria,
Australia; School of Psychological Sciences,
Monash University, Clayton, Victoria, Australia

**STEFANOS N. KALES, MD, MPH, FACP,
FACOEM**
Professor and Director, Occupational Medicine
Residency, Professor of Medicine, Harvard
Medical School, Harvard T.H. Chan School of
Public Health, Boston, Massachusetts, USA;
Division Chief, Occupational Medicine,
Cambridge Health Alliance, Cambridge,
Massachusetts, USA

DAMIEN LÉGER, MD, PhD
Université de Paris, Paris Descartes, EA 7330
VIFASOM (Vigilance Fatigue Sommeil et Santé
Publique), Assistance Publique Hôpitaux de
Paris, APHP-5, Hôtel-Dieu de Paris, Centre du
Sommeil et de la Vigilance, Paris, France

ORESTE MARRONE, MD
Istituto per la Ricerca e l'Innovazione
Biomedica (IRIB), National Research Council
(CNR), Palermo, Italy

CATHERINE A. McCALL, MD
Department of Pulmonary, Critical Care, and
Sleep Medicine, VA Puget Sound Health Care
System, Department of Psychiatry, University
of Washington Sleep Medicine Center, Seattle,
Washington, USA

WALTER T. McNICHOLAS, MD
Newman Professor, School of Medicine,
University College Dublin, Department of
Respiratory and Sleep Medicine, St. Vincent's
Hospital Group, Dublin, Ireland; First Affiliated
Hospital of Guangzhou Medical University,
Guangzhou, China

**JEAN-ARTHUR MICOULAUD-FRANCHI,
MD, PhD**
USR CNRS 3413 SANPSY Sommeil, Addiction
et NeuroPSYchiatrie, SANPSY, USR 3413,
Université Bordeaux, CHU de Bordeaux, Sleep
Clinic, Pôle Neurosciences Cliniques,
Bordeaux, France

MICHAEL A. PARENTEAU, MD, JD, FCLM
Occupational Medicine Resident, Harvard T.H.
Chan School of Public Health, Boston,
Massachusetts, USA

THOMAS PENZEL, Dr rer physiol, Dipl Phys
Professor, Scientific Director, Sleep Medicine
Center, Charité – Universitätsmedizin Berlin,
Berlin, Germany

EMILIE PEPIN, MD
Université de Paris, Paris Descartes, EA 7330
VIFASOM (Vigilance Fatigue Sommeil et Santé
Publique), Assistance Publique Hôpitaux de
Paris, APHP-5, Hôtel-Dieu de Paris, Centre du
Sommeil et de la Vigilance, Paris, France

PIERRE PHILIP, MD, PhD
USR CNRS 3413 SANPSY Sommeil, Addiction
et NeuroPSYchiatrie, SANPSY, USR 3413,
Université Bordeaux, CHU de Bordeaux, Sleep
Clinic, Pôle Neurosciences Cliniques,
Bordeaux, France

DAVID RAINEY, MD, MPH, MEd
Assistant Director, Occupational Medicine
Residency, Instructor of Medicine, Harvard
Medical School, Harvard T.H. Chan School of
Public Health, Boston, Massachusetts, USA;
Physician, Cambridge Health Alliance
Occupational Health, Somerville,
Massachusetts, USA

CHRISTOPH SCHÖBEL, Dr med
Professor, Universitätsmedizin Essen,
Ruhrlandklinik - Westdeutsches
Lungenzentrum, am Universitätsklinikum
Essen gGmbH, Essen, Germany

SHANNON S. SULLIVAN, MD
Medical Director, SleepEval Research Institute,
Palo Alto, California, USA

JACQUES TAILLARD, PhD
USR CNRS 3413 SANPSY Sommeil, Addiction
et NeuroPSYchiatrie, SANPSY, USR 3413,
Université Bordeaux, Bordeaux, France

CHRISTIAN VEAUTHIER, Dr med
Physician, Sleep Medicine Center, Charité –
Universitätsmedizin Berlin, Berlin,
Germany

NATHANIEL F. WATSON, MD, MSc
Department of Neurology, University of
Washington Sleep Medicine Center, Seattle,
Washington, USA

Contents

Sleep-related accidents are a frequent cause of death and injury in the world. Poor sleep hygiene is responsible for sleep deprivation, which is clearly associated with an increased risk of accidents. Evidence shows that self-reported sleepiness at the wheel and reporting of inappropriate line-crossings are strong predictors of accident risk. Although the Epworth sleepiness scale is widely used in clinical practice, it is not the best to evaluate driving risks. Simple questions on the occurrence of near misses and sleepiness at the wheel should be asked systematically to address the issue of fitness to drive.

Driving a vehicle during a night shift increases the accident risk and incidents of falling asleep at the wheel. Individuals having worked a night shift (in any type of occupation) run a similar risk when commuting home from a night shift. Early starts of driving may increase risk. Detailed field studies of sleepiness indicate high levels of sleepiness during late night driving. The mechanism includes exposure to the circadian trough of alertness during work and sleep loss. High levels of sleepiness and sleep loss associated with night and early morning work define the diagnosis of shift work disorder.

Driving while sleepy on a regular basis may be due to sleep restriction associated with work schedules or with poor sleep hygiene. It also may be associated with sleep disorders or with sedative drugs. This review assesses the potential consequences of driving sleepy on a regular basis from a societal point of view. Driving while sleepy on a regular basis increases the risk of motor vehicle accidents (MVAs), impairs the ability to work, has an impact on productivity, and probably also has an impact on the risk of non-MVA occupational accidents and on public disasters.

Obstructive sleep apnea is associated with excessive daytime sleepiness in about 50% of cases, and with increased risk of driving accidents. Treatment with continuous positive airway pressure effectively decreases such risk, but compliance with continuous positive airway pressure treatment is often suboptimal. According to the European Union Directive on driving risk, retention of a driving license in patients with obstructive sleep apnea requires assessment of sleepiness and

adherence to continuous positive airway pressure treatment, but there remains un-
certainty on the optimal methods to assess sleepiness on a large scale.

Many patients with obstructive sleep apnea syndrome (OSAS) drive a vehicle both
for pleasure and as part of their employment. Some, but not all, patients with
OSAS are at increased risk of being involved in road traffic accidents. Clinicians
are often asked to make recommendations about an individual's fitness to drive,
and these are likely to be inconsistent in the absence of objective criteria. This article
discusses the current practice of the assessment of individuals' sleepiness with
respect to driving, the limitations of available techniques, and future possibilities.

Sleep disorders in commercial drivers are common and treatable. Left unidentified,
they lead to a host of adverse consequences, including daytime sleepiness,
adverse health effects, economic costs, and public safety risks owing to
sleepiness-related crashes. The best studied of these is obstructive sleep apnea,
which is common and identifiable among commercial drivers. This article provides
an overview of screening, and specific approaches to screen for and manage
obstructive sleep apnea in commercial drivers with the goal of reducing the risk
of vehicular crashes.

This article reports on sleepiness, drowsiness, tiredness, and fatigue. An assessment of sleepiness can be done with electroencephalograms, electrooculograms,
and electromyograms in validated tests, such as the multiple sleep latency test
and the maintenance of wakefulness test. These 2 tests serve as references for
quantitative assessment of daytime sleepiness and drowsiness. Correlates for
sleepiness, such as reaction time tests, can be used but are less reliable. Questionnaires are self-administered and popular measures for perceived sleepiness. Driver
drowsiness assessment is an important part of sleep laboratory testing, because European Union regulations require assessments due to risk of accidents in patients
with sleep disorders.

Drowsy driving is common and causes 21% of fatal crashes. Individuals at risk
include young men, shift workers, older adults, and people with chronic short sleep
duration, untreated obstructive sleep apnea (OSA), and narcolepsy. Untreated OSA
is a particular concern in commercial drivers, who are at higher risk for the disorder.
Treatment for sleep problems such as sleep extension for chronic short sleep, positive airway pressure (PAP) for OSA, pharmacologic treatments, and drowsy driving
countermeasures may reduce the risk of crashes. Implementing screening measures to identify common sleep problems contributing to drowsy driving continues
to be of high importance.

Sleepiness remains a major contributor to road crashes. Driver monitoring systems identify early signs of sleepiness and alert drivers, using real-time analysis of eyelid movements, EEG activity, and steering control. Other vehicle adaptations warn drivers of lane departures or collision hazards, with higher vehicle automation actively taking over vehicle control to prevent run off the road incidents and institute emergency braking. Similarly, road adaptations warn drivers (rumble strips) or mitigate crash severity (barriers). Infrastructure to encourage drivers to use countermeasures, such as rest stops for napping, is also important. The effectiveness of adaptations varies for different road users.

Sleepiness accounts for approximately 20% of major highway motor vehicle accidents (MVAs) and the most common medical disorder associated with sleepiness is obstructive sleep apnea (OSA). OSA patients are 2 to 3 times more likely to have an MVA than the general population, although continuous positive airway pressure therapy can remove this excess risk. Several jurisdictions have introduced regulations to limit driving in patients with moderate or severe OSA associated with sleepiness until the disorder is effectively treated. Successful implementation of such regulations requires education regarding risk-benefit relationships of relevant stakeholders, including patients, clinicians, and employers in the transportation industry.

Human fatigue is an important factor in transportation safety and a major causal factor of accidents. Employers play a vital role in minimizing fatigue-related risk, and are legally liable for damages arising from failure to address the risk. By taking an active role as stakeholders in transportation safety, employers not only reduce their risk of adverse safety events and limit their legal liability but may also benefit from improvements in productivity, morale, and health care expenditures. Employers should focus on reducing fatigue-related risk, with ongoing support from sleep safety research.

Preface

Sleep Disturbances and Disorders: A Poorly Recognized Accident Risk

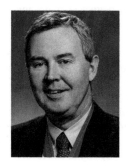

Walter T. McNicholas, MD
Editor

Speed and alcohol consumption are widely recognized contributory factors to motor vehicle accidents (MVA) and are almost universally regulated throughout the world by speed limits and blood/urine/breath alcohol levels while driving. In recent decades, there has been growing recognition that sleep disturbances and disorders with consequent sleepiness during the waking hours also represent important contributing factors to driving accident risk.[1] However, this risk is difficult to quantify by objective measures such as are employed for speed and alcohol, which inevitably result in sleepiness being a less well-documented contributing factor to MVA. Nonetheless, driving while sleepy confers a similar increased accident risk as driving with a blood alcohol level above the legal limit for most countries. Various reports estimate that sleepiness represents a major contributing factor in about 20% of serious MVA and is particularly likely to be a major factor in MVA on major highways where monotonous driving at relatively high speed is common.[2]

Fatigue and sleepiness because of sleep dysfunction are most common in circumstances of poor sleep hygiene where the affected individual spends too little time in bed and/or experiences disturbed sleep due to poor lifestyle habits. Specific medical disorders may also contribute to sleep disturbance, the most important of which is obstructive sleep apnea (OSA).

OSA is widely reported to increase MVA risk 2- to 3-fold, but this increased risk is removed by effective treatment, which underlines the practical importance of recognition and treatment.[3] Indeed, several jurisdictions have introduced regulations that preclude untreated patients with moderate or severe OSA associated with sleepiness from driving unless effectively treated.[4,5]

The present issue of *Sleep Medicine Clinics* is devoted to the topic of Sleep and Driving and provides a comprehensive review of all aspects of this relationship. Topics discussed include the impact on driving safety of sleep restriction, sleep hygiene, and shift work, in addition to the economic burden of sleepy drivers. The role of OSA in MVA risk is extensively discussed, including the role of screening, effective treatment, and the role of government regulation. The assessment of sleepiness in drivers is an important practical topic, as current limitations in techniques to assess sleepiness limit the ability to objectively measure this factor, and future possibilities, especially technology related, are reviewed. Vehicle and highway adaptations to compensate for sleepy drivers are of increasing importance in promoting driving safety. While these measures are directed at all drivers, they have special relevance to the sleepy driver. The role of the employer in screening for sleep disorders among professional drivers is also discussed as there is growing evidence that targeted screening of truck drivers for disorders such as

Sleep Med Clin 14 (2019) xiii–xiv
https://doi.org/10.1016/j.jsmc.2019.08.008
1556-407X/19/© 2019 Published by Elsevier Inc.

sleep.theclinics.com

OSA confers financial benefits to the industry as well as improved highway safety.[6]

Walter T. McNicholas, MD
School of Medicine
University College Dublin
Department of Respiratory and
Sleep Medicine
St. Vincent's Hospital Group
Merrion Road, Dublin 4, Ireland

First Affiliated Hospital of
Guangzhou Medical University
Guangzhou, China

E-mail address:
walter.mcnicholas@ucd.ie

REFERENCES

1. Bioulac S, Franchi J-AM, Arnaud M, et al. Risk of motor vehicle accidents related to sleepiness at the wheel: a systematic review and meta-analysis. Sleep 2018;41(7).

2. Czeisler CA, Wickwire EM, Barger LK, et al. Sleep-deprived motor vehicle operators are unfit to drive: a multidisciplinary expert consensus statement on drowsy driving. Sleep Health 2016;2(2):94–9.

3. Tregear S, Reston J, Schoelles K, et al. Continuous positive airway pressure reduces risk of motor vehicle crash among drivers with obstructive sleep apnea: systematic review and meta-analysis. Sleep 2010; 33(10):1373–80.

4. Bonsignore MR, Randerath W, Riha R, et al. New rules on driver licensing for patients with obstructive sleep apnea: European Union Directive 2014/85/EU. J Sleep Res 2016;25(1):3–4.

5. McNicholas WT, Rodenstein D. Sleep apnoea and driving risk: the need for regulation. Eur Respir Rev 2015;24(138):602–6.

6. Burks SV, Anderson JE, Bombyk M, et al. Nonadherence with employer-mandated sleep apnea treatment and increased risk of serious truck crashes. Sleep 2016;39(5):967–75.

Sleep Restriction, Sleep Hygiene, and Driving Safety

The Importance of Situational Sleepiness

Pierre Philip, MD, PhD[a,b,c],*, Jacques Taillard, PhD[a,b], Jean-Arthur Micoulaud-Franchi, MD, PhD[a,b,c]

KEYWORDS

- Sleepiness • Driving accident • Sleep restriction • Sleep hygiene

KEY POINTS

- Chronic sleep restriction impacts drivers in developed countries.
- Sleepiness at the wheel is a better predictor of accident risk than the Epworth sleepiness scale.
- Inappropriate line crossings are strong warnings of future sleep-related accidents.
- Road safety campaigns should address not only acute but also chronic sleep deprivation all year long.

INTRODUCTION

Traffic accidents are an increasing cause of death and injury in the world, initially in western societies but now more and more in the developing countries.[1] Although the passive safety of vehicles has increased enormously, human behaviors frequently remain inappropriate for safe driving. Many countries have launched road safety campaigns in recent decades to decrease mortality and morbidity on their roads. Alcohol and excessive speed are known to be major killers, and the health status of drivers is now receiving attention as a cause of accidents. Sleepiness at the wheel is clearly associated with an increased risk of accidents.[2] Extended or nocturnal driving is associated with accidents, but few studies have differentiated fatigue, which is usually seen as being caused by long driving time and sleepiness, which is cause by reduced sleep, extended time awake,

and/or being awake at the circadian trough.[3,4] Sleep hygiene is also a key issue to explain sleep-related accidents.[2] This article examines the definition of sleepiness to predict accident risk, mainly in terms of sleep hygiene and the chronobiological determinants of traffic accidents. However, sleep apnea syndrome is also associated with traffic accidents and other diseases such as insomnia and narcolepsy.[4]

Although both the European Union and the United States have launched public campaigns to make their citizens aware of the risk of drowsy driving (eg, the US National Sleep Foundation "Drive Alert–Arrive Alive" campaign, "Wake Up Bus" in Europe), the identification of specific drivers at risk of or behaviors increasing risk of traffic accidents remains a problem. This article presents an update on the relationship between sleep restriction and traffic accidents and

Disclosure Statement: None to declared.
[a] USR CNRS 3413 SANPSY Sommeil, Addiction et NeuroPSYchiatrie, Bordeaux, France; [b] SANPSY, USR 3413, Université Bordeaux, CHU de Bordeaux, Place Amelie Raba Leon, Bordeaux 33000, France; [c] Sleep Clinic, CHU de Bordeaux, Pôle Neurosciences Cliniques, Bordeaux, France
* Corresponding author. SANPSY, USR 3413, CHU de Bordeaux, 13éme étage Pellegrin, Place Amelie Raba Leon, Bordeaux 33000, France.
E-mail address: Pr.philip@free.fr

Sleep Med Clin 14 (2019) 407–412
https://doi.org/10.1016/j.jsmc.2019.07.002

underlines the importance of the definition of sleepiness to address the exact risk of this symptom.

PHYSIOLOGIC FACTORS MODULATING SLEEPINESS

Sleepiness is a complex symptom that may be confused with fatigue. Technically, sleepiness occurs when chronobiological or homeostatic sleep pressure increases to force the brain to go from a state of arousal to a state of sleep. Alerting systems are then stimulated and somewhat prevent the occurrence of sleep.

The first and most common factor involved in sleepiness is extended wakefulness or sleep deprivation, which significantly increases homeostatic pressure and generates excessive daytime sleepiness. The homeostatic drive is regulated by the release of adenosine, which fixes to specific brain receptors. The amount of these receptors is genetically determined and variable between subjects.[5,6]

Sleepiness is also driven by the circadian system, which is controlled in part by the suprachiasmatic nucleus located in the hypothalamus and is entrained/synchronized essentially by the light/dark cycle. It generates circadian rhythms that dip and rise at different times of the day. It imposes the timing of periods of sleepiness during the night and wakefulness during the day.[7] In adults, the strongest wake drive occurs in the early evening prior to the onset of the nocturnal sleep period and has been called the "forbidden zone for sleep." The strongest sleep drive occurs in the early morning prior to the onset of the diurnal wake period.[8] Cognitive performance remains stable during a usual waking day (approximately 17 h of wakefulness) and then declines during the usual nighttime after midnight, with the maximum decrement occurring near the 24th hour of wakefulness, that is, the early morning.[9]

QUANTIFYING SLEEPINESS: DIFFERENCES BETWEEN NEUTRAL AND "AT RISK" SLEEPINESS

Sleepiness can be defined as a subjective perception or as an objective measure via electrophysiological measurements. The Stanford Sleepiness Scale (SSS)[10] and the Karolinska Scale[11] have been used in many sleep deprivation protocols and in healthy subjects. They measure instantaneous sleepiness via straightforward questions. Because they focus on a short period of time, they hardly reflect the mean level of sleepiness over days or weeks; yet these data are required to quantify the impact of poor sleep hygiene.

Behavioral scales were developed in the 1990s to quantify sleepiness. Their rationale was to explore specific activities or periods of the day that could promote sleepiness. The Epworth Sleepiness Scale (ESS)[12] is the most famous and combines stimulant and passive conditions (eg, "How likely are you to doze off or fall asleep" during "watching TV" versus "sitting and talking to someone?"). Its authors wanted to capture the average amount of sleepiness to which patients are exposed. It was also an ingenious way to reproduce clinical evaluation over long periods of time (ie, a few weeks) in order to quantify the positive impact of the treatment of sleep disorders. However, regarding accident risk, these scales tend to provide composite scores that do not reflect the inability to remain awake or how easy it is to fall asleep in nonstimulating conditions.

There is a great need for scales able to quantify "at risk" sleepiness, especially in the context of driving, which concerns millions of adults worldwide. Accident risk is the result of a cognitive inability to pursue driving because of the onset of sleepiness. It is therefore important to use situational scales to better quantify the severity of excessive daytime sleepiness in the precise situation where the subject is exposed to the risk. Considering the predictive value of accident risk, results obtained with the ESS have been contradictory. For example, Connor[13] found a strong correlation between SSS scores and accident risk but no relationship between chronic sleepiness and traffic accidents. Other authors[4,14] found a relationship between ESS scores and the risk of traffic accidents among nonprofessional drivers. More importantly, professional drivers had to reach a severe level of sleepiness before reporting a real accident risk, so ESS scores rendered more of a binary yes/no evaluation with a cutoff above 16 than a progressive measure of accident risk.

Conscious of the issues related to the shortcomings of the ESS, Hobson and colleagues[15] developed a specific variant of the scale in order to better predict accident risk in a specific group of parkinsonian patients. The scale results from the combination of the ESS and the Inappropriate Sleep Composite Score (ISCS), a scale consisting of 4 items that allows assessment of sleep propensity in situations where it is particularly unusual to fall asleep, such as driving, eating a meal, working, and doing housework. The items are scored from 0 to 3 and are summed. The validity of the Hobson variant regarding the impact on everyday functioning shows that it predicts accident risk better than the ESS. However, it has only been used for patients with Parkinson disease on dopamine agonists.

A meta-analysis published in 2017[16] provided new perspectives to evaluate the "at-risk" dimension of excessive daytime sleepiness in a robust simple way. A single question is asked about the propensity to fall asleep in an inappropriate situation, particularly an at-risk one such as driving. After a systematic review of the different ways of evaluating sleepiness at the wheel, the authors suggested that the following question: "Have you experienced in the previous year at least one episode of severe sleepiness at the wheel that made driving difficult or forced you to stop the car?" was optimal to predict the accident risk associated with driving. They found that sleepiness at the wheel was associated with a mean increased risk of motor vehicle accidents (pooled odds ratio [OR] 2.51 [95% confidence interval (CI) 1.87; 3.39]) in a sample of more than 50,000 participants.

SLEEP HYGIENE AND DRIVING RISK
Rest/Activity Patterns

Nonprofessional drivers
In the 1990s, Philip and colleagues[17] conducted a series of studies investigating the role of sleep deprivation and sleepiness at the wheel among large populations of highway drivers. At that time when air conditioning was not widespread in automobiles in Europe, public health campaigns recommended leaving early in the morning or late at night to avoid heat and traffic jams. A first study demonstrated that time of departure was closely related to sleep restriction and that sleep-related episodes at the wheel were quite frequent in this population of drivers. Several publications over a 20-year period accumulated more evidence about the link between sleep hygiene and accident risks, not only in summertime drivers, but also in drivers on the highway all year long.[4,18,19] Other groups in different countries (United States, New Zealand) confirmed the importance of sleep deprivation or nocturnal driving in the occurrence of sleep-related accidents.[13,20]

Experimental studies have shown the impact of sleep deprivation or extended wakefulness on real driving performances[21] in healthy subjects. Vakulin and colleagues[22] tested in untreated obstructive sleep apnea (OSA) subjects the impact of sleep deprivation compared with a control group of healthy subjects during a driving simulation task. Patients with OSA crashed more frequently than control participants (1 vs 24 participants; OR, 25.4; $P = .03$) and crashed more frequently after sleep restriction (OR, 4.0; $P<.01$) than after normal sleep. Braking reaction time was also slower after sleep restriction than after normal sleep. More recently, Gottlieb and colleagues[23] used a large cohort to confirm the relative impact of restricted sleep and positive apnea/hypopnea index to predict accidental risk. Sleeping 6 hours per night was associated with a 33% increased crash risk, compared with sleeping 7 or 8 hours per night. These associations were present even in those who did not report excessive sleepiness. The population-attributable fraction of motor vehicle crashes was 10% due to sleep apnea and 9% due to sleep duration less than 7 hours. These results demonstrate that OSA patients should be careful regarding their sleep hygiene.

Although a major focus in the 1990s was the association of acute sleep deprivation and nocturnal driving, profound societal changes in recent years have significantly changed sleep-wake patterns. The advent of the smartphone and social networks has increased nocturnal and 24/7 activities. Several studies in the United States and Europe have thrown light on what constitutes mean sleep duration. As incredible as it may seem, it was not until 1995 that general recommendations on mean sleep duration in adult and infant populations were published.[24] Adults should sleep between 7 and 9 hours and never less than 7 hours. Although the US data might be considered as reassuring regarding chronic sleep deprivation,[25] the situation in Europe is somewhat different. Quera Salva published an article showing a reduction in sleep over a 15-year period among French drivers.[26] They found that usual sleep duration decreased among French drivers between 1996 and 2011. Interestingly, this reduction was associated with an increase in sleepiness as measured by the ESS. The number of drivers with an ESS score above 15 increased 2.5-fold over the 15-year period. Not only behavioral but also situational sleepiness increased over time. Sleepiness forcing the driver to stop driving increased from 5.6% in 1996 to 14% in 2014.

More recently and still in France, Leger and colleagues showed in a large representative sample of the French population (n = 12,370) that sleep deprivation was growing with a mean sleep duration under 7 hours of sleep.[27] Thirty-eight percent of the sample reported suffering from a sleep debt at night. This finding should be related to behavioral changes explaining sleep-related accidents. Driving is frequently associated with extensive wakefulness, which induces sleepiness at the wheel. Studying large populations of drivers, the authors demonstrated that long-distance driving was frequently associated with sleep curtailment. Extensive wakefulness is also associated with nocturnal driving, which alters driving performances and leads to highway line crossings.

Inappropriate line crossings are strong predictors of accidental risk.[28]

Many studies have assessed the predictive value of self-reported sleepiness at the wheel and the predictive value of the driving risk. In a meta-analysis, Bioulac and colleagues[16] analyzed 10 cross-sectional studies (51,520 participants), 6 case-control studies (4904 participants), and 1 cohort study (13,674 participants) to evaluate the danger of self-reported sleepiness at the wheel. Sleepiness at the wheel was associated with an increased risk of motor vehicle accidents (pooled OR 2.51 [95% CI 1.87; 3.39]). A significant heterogeneity was found between the individual risk estimates (Q = 93.21; I2 = 83%), possibly because of the different definitions used in the studies. The authors therefore recommended using the specific question "Have you experienced in the previous year at least 1 episode of severe sleepiness at the wheel that made driving difficult or forced you to stop the car?"

Professional drivers

Sleep deprivation affects not only the general population of automobile drivers but also many professional drivers worldwide. A study of professional truck drivers[29] demonstrated a mean duration of sleep of 4.78 h/d in a 5-day period. Fifty-six percent of drivers presented at least 6 noncontinuous minutes of electroencephalographic (EEG)-recorded sleep while driving. The vast majority of these microsleep episodes occurred during the late night and early morning. Interestingly, the episodes of sleep at the wheel were not associated with accidents, so actual sleep at the wheel in trained professionals does not necessarily mean an accident in 100% of cases. A possible explanation is that automatic behaviors allow drivers to remain on the road when they sleep lightly for very brief periods.[29] Nevertheless, sleep restriction is dangerous and involves a significant driving risk for most drivers. More recently, Sunwoo and colleagues[30] performed a cross-sectional study comparing sleep habits and sleep problems in 110 truck drivers with 1001 matched controls from the general population of South Korea. Multivariate regression analysis was performed to determine whether commercial vehicle (CMV) drivers were independently associated with these sleep problems compared with controls. As found in other publications, the prevalence of high OSA and insomnia was high with 35.5% and 15.2%, respectively, which was significantly higher than the 12.2% and 4.1% found in controls, respectively (P<.001 for both). Although CMV drivers had higher ESS scores than controls, the prevalence of daytime sleepiness did not differ between the 2 groups (19.1% vs 16.8%, P = .54). After adjusting for covariates, CMV drivers had 3.68-fold higher odds (95% CI 2.29–5.84) of having OSA and 2.97-fold higher odds (95% CI, 1.46–6.06) of suffering from insomnia compared with controls. However, the degree of daytime sleepiness was not independently associated with CMV drivers. The prevalence of OSA and insomnia in CMV drivers was higher than that in the general population. Daytime sleepiness was associated with increased body mass index (BMI), depression, OSA, and short sleep duration, which confirm the strong links between sleep hygiene and excessive daytime sleepiness in this specific population. Interestingly, OSA is common in professional drivers, because of their high BMI and the fact that many are middle-aged men.

Shiftwork, Time on Task, and Driving

Cognitive performance remained stable during a usual waking day (for approximately 17 h of wakefulness) and then declined during the usual nighttime (after midnight), with the maximum decrement occurring near the 24th hour of wakefulness (early morning).[9,31] The risk of accidents related to sleepiness or man-caused catastrophes is greater during the night and especially between 3 a.m. and 5 a.m. than during the day,[32] hence the notion of black times.[33] Barger and colleagues[34] conducted a prospective nationwide, Web-based survey in which 2737 residents in their first postgraduate year (interns) completed 17,003 monthly reports that provided detailed information about work hours, work shifts of an extended duration, documented motor vehicle crashes, near-miss incidents, and incidents involving involuntary sleeping. The odds ratios for reporting a motor vehicle crash and for reporting a near-miss incident after an extended work shift, as compared with a shift that was not of extended duration, were 2.3 and 5.9, respectively. In a prospective analysis, every extended work shift that was scheduled in a month increased the monthly risk of a motor vehicle crash by 9.1% and increased the monthly risk of a crash during the commute from work by 16.2%. In months in which interns worked 5 or more extended shifts, the risk that they would fall asleep while driving or while stopped in traffic was significantly increased (ORs, 2.39 and 3.69 respectively).

The same team in a more recent real driving study[3] showed that participants tested after daytime work and after a nightshift had a significantly higher rate of lane excursions, blink duration, and number of slow eye movements during postnight shift drives compared with postsleep drives. This performance decrement can be related to the circadian phase but also to the cumulative effect of workload and sleep pressure. Time on task is an additive risk, and the authors showed that extensive nocturnal driving dramatically worsens driving performance. Eight hours of nocturnal driving increased sixfold the number of inappropriate highway line crossings compared with a 2-h nocturnal driving session (3–5 a.m.).[21] These results suggest that fatigue related to driving duration is amplified at night, so maximal driving duration should be shorter at night than during the day.

Sleep duration, work duration, time on task, and shift work schedules are key factors to control to reduce behavioral sleepiness at the wheel. As described previously in the conceptual approach to situational sleepiness, one cannot rule out the importance of economic constraints in professional drivers and self-reported sleepiness at the wheel. Objective evaluation of excessive daytime sleepiness via the Maintenance of Wakefulness Test can be a good strategy in this setting.

FUTURE CONSIDERATIONS

Although much has already been done in this field, many questions remain unanswered. At the diagnostic level there is still no simple objective measure to quantify the risk to drivers, unlike other accident risk factors that can be easily assessed, such as by using a breathalyzer for alcohol testing. Ideally, one need a somnotest to quantify the driving risk, but up to now driving simulators or electroencephalogram (EEG) measures have provided only indirect and variable estimations of the driving risk and are obviously not practicable for use outside the clinic or laboratory. Connected car technologies might be the future to evaluate drivers' behaviors.

A growing body of evidence is showing that self-reported sleepiness at the wheel and the reporting of inappropriate line-crossings are strong predictors of accident risk. These 2 questions should be systematically asked when addressing the issue of fitness to drive. While the ESS is widely used in clinical practice, it is not the best scale to evaluate driving risks.[16]

The impact of extensive driving is also a key factor in the research agenda because of the high prevalence of sleep deprivation in professional drivers, especially in the United States, where they are paid by miles driven. After addressing the issues of acute sleep deprivation, one also needs to consider sleep hygiene in the longer term. Road safety campaigns on the risks of chronic sleep deprivation and drowsy driving need to be released in every country.

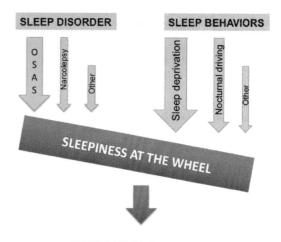

Fig. 1. Sleepiness at the wheel as common final pathway to evaluate risk of motor vehicle accidents.

It is also important to consider that poor sleep hygiene not only affects healthy drivers, but may occur in patients suffering from sleep disorders like OSA (**Fig. 1**). Because of the large prevalence of these patients, they should be educated to the same standards as healthy drivers.

Defining at-risk phenotypes regarding situational sleepiness is probably the next step in order to personalize safety campaigns. The use of health technologies to monitor sleep hygiene could help achieve this goal.

REFERENCES

1. Lagarde E. Road traffic injury is an escalating burden in Africa and deserves proportionate research efforts. PLoS Med 2007;4(6):e170.
2. Connor J, Whitlock G, Norton R, et al. The role of driver sleepiness in car crashes: a systematic review of epidemiological studies. Accid Anal Prev 2001; 33(1):31–41.
3. Lee ML, Howard ME, Horrey WJ, et al. High risk of near-crash driving events following night-shift work. Proc Natl Acad Sci U S A 2016;113(1):176–81.
4. Philip P, Sagaspe P, Lagarde E, et al. Sleep disorders and accidental risk in a large group of regular registered highway drivers. Sleep Med 2010; 11(10):973–9.
5. Retey JV, Adam M, Honegger E, et al. A functional genetic variation of adenosine deaminase affects the duration and intensity of deep sleep in humans. Proc Natl Acad Sci U S A 2005;102(43):15676–81.
6. Retey JV, Adam M, Gottselig JM, et al. Adenosinergic mechanisms contribute to individual differences in sleep deprivation-induced changes in neurobehavioral function and brain rhythmic activity. J Neurosci 2006;26(41):10472–9.

7. Czeisler CA, Weitzman E, Moore-Ede MC, et al. Human sleep: its duration and organization depend on its circadian phase. Science 1980;210(4475):1264–7.

8. Lavie P. Ultrashort sleep-waking schedule. III. "Gates" and "forbidden zones" for sleep. Electroencephalogr Clin Neurophysiol 1986;63:414–25.

9. Taillard J, Philip P, Claustrat B, et al. Time course of neurobehavioral alertness during extended wakefulness in morning- and evening-type healthy sleepers. Chronobiol Int 2011;28(6):520–7.

10. Hoddes E, Dement WC, Zarcone V. The development and use of the Stanford sleepiness scale (SSS). Psychophysiology 1972;9:150.

11. Gillberg M, Kecklund G, Akerstedt T. Relations between performance and subjective ratings of sleepiness during a night awake. Sleep 1994;17(3): 236–41.

12. Johns MW. A new method for measuring daytime sleepiness: the Epworth sleepiness scale. Sleep 1991;14(6):540–5.

13. Connor J, Norton R, Ameratunga S, et al. Driver sleepiness and risk of serious injury to car occupants: population based case control study. BMJ 2002;324(7346):1125.

14. Howard ME, Desai AV, Grunstein RR, et al. Sleepiness, sleep-disordered breathing, and accident risk factors in commercial vehicle drivers. Am J Respir Crit Care Med 2004;170(9):1014–21.

15. Hobson DE, Lang AE, Martin WR, et al. Excessive daytime sleepiness and sudden-onset sleep in Parkinson disease: a survey by the Canadian Movement Disorders Group. JAMA 2002;287(4):455–63.

16. Bioulac S, Franchi JM, Arnaud M, et al. Risk of motor vehicle accidents related to sleepiness at the wheel: a systematic review and meta-analysis. Sleep 2017; 40(10).

17. Philip P, Ghorayeb I, Stoohs R, et al. Determinants of sleepiness in automobile drivers. J Psychosom Res 1996;41:279–88.

18. Philip P, Taillard J, Gilleminault C, et al. Long distance driving and self-induced sleep deprivation among automobile drivers. Sleep 1999;22:475–80.

19. Sagaspe P, Taillard J, Bayon V, et al. Sleepiness, near-misses and driving accidents among a representative population of French drivers. J Sleep Res 2010;19(4):578–84.

20. Sagberg F. Road accidents caused by drivers falling asleep. Accid Anal Prev 1999;31(6):639–49.

21. Sagaspe P, Taillard J, Akerstedt T, et al. Extended driving impairs nocturnal driving performances. PLoS One 2008;3(10):e3493.

22. Vakulin A, Baulk SD, Catcheside PG, et al. Effects of alcohol and sleep restriction on simulated driving performance in untreated patients with obstructive sleep apnea. Ann Intern Med 2009;151(7):447–55.

23. Gottlieb DJ, Ellenbogen JM, Bianchi MT, et al. Sleep deficiency and motor vehicle crash risk in the general population: a prospective cohort study. BMC Med 2018;16(1):44.

24. Watson NF, Badr MS, Belenky G, et al. Joint consensus statement of the American Academy of Sleep Medicine and Sleep Research Society on the recommended amount of sleep for a healthy adult: methodology and discussion. Sleep 2015; 38(8):1161–83.

25. Basner M, Dinges DF. Sleep duration in the United States 2003-2016: first signs of success in the fight against sleep deficiency? Sleep 2018;41(4).

26. Quera-Salva MA, Hartley S, Sauvagnac-Quera R, et al. Association between reported sleep need and sleepiness at the wheel: comparative study on French highways between 1996 and 2011. BMJ Open 2016;6(12):e012382.

27. Leger D, Zeghnoun K, Richard JB, et al. Prevalence and sociodemographics associated with total sleep time in France and insomnia in 12370 individuals. Sleep 2019;42(Suppl 1):A169–70.

28. Philip P, Chaufton C, Taillard J, et al. Maintenance of wakefulness test scores and driving performance in sleep disorder patients and controls. Int J Psychophysiol 2013;89(2):195–202.

29. Mitler MM, Miller JC, Lipsitz JJ, et al. The sleep of long-haul truck drivers. N Engl J Med 1997; 337(11):755–61.

30. Sunwoo JS, Shin DS, Hwangbo Y, et al. High risk of obstructive sleep apnea, insomnia, and daytime sleepiness among commercial motor vehicle drivers. Sleep Breath 2019. [Epub ahead of print].

31. Dijk DJ, Duffy JF, Czeisler CA. Circadian and sleep/wake dependent aspects of subjective alertness and cognitive performance. J Sleep Res 1992;1(2): 112–7.

32. Reinberg A, Smolensky MH, Riedel M, et al. Chronobiologic perspectives of black time–Accident risk is greatest at night: an opinion paper. Chronobiol Int 2015;32(7):1005–18.

33. Folkard S. Black times: temporal determinants of transport safety. Accid Anal Prev 1997;29:417–30.

34. Barger LK, Cade BE, Ayas NT, et al. Extended work shifts and the risk of motor vehicle crashes among interns. N Engl J Med 2005;352(2):125–34.

Shift Work – Sleepiness and Sleep in Transport

Torbjörn Åkerstedt, PhD

KEYWORDS

• Sleep • Sleepiness • Fatigue • Night • Duration • Driving

KEY POINTS

- Driving a vehicle during a night shift increases the accident risk and incidents of falling asleep at the wheel.
- Individuals having worked a night shift (in any type of occupation) run a similar risk when commuting home from a night shift.
- Early starts of driving may increase risk.
- Detailed field studies of sleepiness indicate high levels of sleepiness during late night driving.
- The mechanism includes exposure to the circadian trough of alertness during work and sleep loss.
- High levels of sleepiness and sleep loss associated with night and early morning work define the diagnosis of Shift Work Disorder.
- Interventions or treatment to mitigate sleep and fatigue problems in shift work are rarely implemented.

INTRODUCTION

A recent meta-analysis shows that sleepiness at the wheel is clearly linked to road crashes, with an odds ratio (OR) of 2.5.[1] The main causes are suggested to be sleep disorders (particularly sleep apnea), sleep deprivation, and shift work. Another recent review also finds working shifts (with night work) a common cause of sleep-related crashes.[2] This article will focus on shift work, and particularly, such work in the transport sector.

Before looking at the effects of shift work, there is need for a short introduction on what is meant by shift work. Shift work is a rather imprecise concept, but usually refers to a work hour system in which a relay of employees extends the period of production beyond the conventional daytime third of the 24-h cycle. Four major types may be discerned: day work, permanently displaced work hours, rotating shift work, and roster work. Day work involves work periods that fall between approximately 7 a.m. and 7 p.m. Permanently displaced work hours require the individual to work either a morning shift (approximately 6 a.m. to 2 p.m.), an afternoon shift (approximately 2 to 10 p.m.), or a night shift (approximately 10 p.m. to 5 a.m.). Rotating shift work involves alternation between shifts, either all 3 shifts (3-shift work) or 2 shifts (2-shift work). The latter usually involves the morning plus the afternoon shift. Three-shift work is often subdivided according to the number of teams that are used to cover the 24 hours - usually 3 to 6 teams. A higher number of teams is required for rapidly rotating schedules. Roster work is similar to rotating shift work but may be less regular, more flexible, and less geared to specific teams. The roster shifts are mainly determined by the needs of production being different at different times of day. This is in contrast to traditional shift work, where the rate of production is constant across the 24 hours. Roster work is seldom used in industry but rather in transport, health care, law enforcement, and news media.

The author reports no conflicts of interest.
Department of Clinical Neuroscience, Karolinska Institute, Stress Research Institute, Stockholm University, Nobels vag 9, Stockholm 17177, Sweden
E-mail address: torbjorn.akerstedt@ki.se

The reason for shift work being of interest in relation to sleepy driving and accident risk is that work during the night will not only prevent sleep, but also expose the worker to night time circadian trough and to an extended time awake. This will result in sleepiness during the night work hours (eg, truck drivers). However, a night spent working also means that the worker is exposed to sleepiness while driving home from a night shift, regardless of whether he or she is a truck driver. Finally, shifts that start early (morning shifts) will interfere at least partially with normal sleep hours.

ACCIDENT, OR FALLING ASLEEP, STUDIES

The reason the considerable interest in shiftwork in transport is the accident risk linked to sleepy driving. Case control studies have shown shift work is common among those who have been involved in a crash.[3,4] The OR in the Stutts and colleagues study was greater than 14 for night work and greater than 3 for other, which included rotating shift work. Night work had the largest F-ratio among several background variables, including sleep duration less than 5h and various sleep problems. The strongest predictor, however, was Epworth Sleepiness Scale (ESS) ratings greater than 16, with an OR greater than 17.

In another case control study, Connor and colleagues[5] interviewed individuals who recently had been involved in a car accident (with hospital visit) on a specific road, compared to others driving on that road, but without having an accident. The results showed that night driving (between 2 and 5 a.m.) had an OR of greater than 5, while retrospective sleepiness ratings from before a crash showed a high OR greater than 8 for higher sleepiness on the Stanford Sleepiness scale (score 4–7), compared to drivers who had been interviewed without having been involved in a crash. Prior sleep of more than 5 hours had an OR of greater than 2. Being a shift worker was not a significant predictor; neither was sleep apnea or habitual sleepiness.

Crummy and colleagues[6] carried out a somewhat similar study. They interviewed 112 injured drivers and found that 50% had at least 1 sleep-related risk factor; 20% had at least 2 risk factors. Being a shift worker, driving at night, and reporting high sleepiness (Karolinska Sleepiness Scale [KSS] >5) were related to sleep-related accidents.

Another interesting outcome is reports of having fallen asleep at the wheel.[7] With respect to post-night shift sleepiness, house staff reports having fallen asleep at a red light (44%), and when driving home (23%) post call, which is 4 times as frequent an amount as in colleagues not being on call. Twenty-eight percent had been involved in motor vehicle accidents (11% for non-on call colleagues).[8] This type of post-call or post-night shift accident risk has been seen in other studies.[9–11]

Harris[12] and Hamelin[13] and Langlois and colleagues[14] used accident statistics and demonstrated that single vehicle truck accidents have, by far, the greatest probability of occurring at night (early morning). Single vehicle accidents are thought to contain a high proportion of sleepiness. The authors carried out a similar study for all types of vehicles in Swedish national accident registers and found an increase in the early morning hours for all types of driving accidents (eg, single, rear-end, heads-on collisions), except for those caused by overtaking.[15] The risk at that time is increased 5.5 times for all types of accidents, 11 times for single vehicle accidents, and 10 times for accidents leading to death. Young age increases risk several times, and male gender doubles the risk.[16]

FIELD STUDIES DESCRIBING SLEEPINESS DURING SHIFT WORK

To understand the role of sleepiness in road accidents, one also needs to investigate in field studies the occurrence of sleepiness, and its relation to work hours. One approach has been to employ long-term video recording of the faces of professional drivers and of the traffic situation. Such recordings are scored for signs of drowsiness, like long-duration eye blinks, closed eyelids, nodding head movements, and similar events. The results suggest inattention, frequently caused by sleepiness, to be the most prevalent cause of near accidents,[17,18] but work hours were not addressed in those studies. Mitler and colleagues,[19] however, made video recordings of long-haul truck drivers on their night and day trips, and found that 6.7% of all 6-minute sections of the recordings showed drowsiness across all types of work hours. The incidence was highest during night driving (11.6%) and lowest during day driving (1.5%).

Mitler and colleagues also recorded electroencephalography (EEG) and electrooculography (EOG), but found few cases of stage 1 sleep, although slow rolling eye movements occurred more frequently. In another EEG study of night driving, increased theta (4-8 Hz) EEG activity and alpha (8–12 Hz) EEG activity were observed during the late night, but not during day driving.[20] Also subjective sleepiness was increased during night driving and was highly correlated with alpha activity.

Pylkkönen and colleagues[21] restricted themselves to sleepiness ratings (KSS)[22] during drives of long-haul truck drivers and found that severe sleepiness (≥7) in 37.8% of drivers on the first night drive of the work week (much lower on the second night drive), and 10% of drivers on morning drives. No other field studies of real night shift driving seem to have been carried out, but train drivers also show a gradual increase in alpha power density and in subjective sleepiness during night driving.[23]

For lack of more studies of professional night shift driving, one may turn to experimental studies of nonprofessionals being asked to drive at night. In this type of study also subjective ratings are carried out frequently, and events like lateral variability and line crossing are also measured as indicators of erratic driving. In 1 such study, 18 participants drove during the night/early morning for 90 minutes on a motorway. Eight participants (42%) had to be taken off the road prematurely, because the driving inspector in the front right seat judged their driving as showing dangerous sleepiness.[24] This group was characterized by increased subjective sleepiness (>8 on the KSS) during the minutes before being stopped. They also showed increases in blink duration, EEG indicators of sleep/sleepiness, and number of line crossings. A clear time on task effect was observed within 20 minutes after start. In this study, no intake of caffeine or similar drugs was permitted during the night, nor napping. It was concluded that late night driving led to dangerous levels of sleepiness in a large proportion of the drivers, and almost as high levels in the rest of the drivers. Similar increases of physiologic and subjective sleepiness, as well as line crossings during late night driving, have been observed in 3 other on-the-road studies.[25–27]

Driving on a closed track is probably different from driving in real traffic, but during a 2-hour drive with 16 nurses on a closed track after a night shift,[28] lane excursions, blink durations, number of slow eye movements, number of premature terminations (for safety reasons), and near crashes increased. Perrier and colleagues[29] saw increased alpha and theta activity, as well as lateral variability during day driving after a night awake compared with driving during the day after a full night's sleep.

To investigate the consistency of the pattern of sleepiness during night driving across studies, the author and colleagues collected a set of driving studies using KSS measures and compared them.[24] KSS increased from approximately 5.5 to 7 units across 50 minutes, and the standard deviation across studies was approximately 0.6 units (ie, the studies were quite homogenous) (**Fig. 1**). The daytime driving showed a similar increase over time, with a starting point around

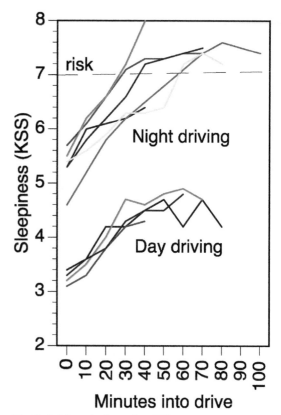

Fig. 1. Driving studies using KSS measures.

KSS = 3.2. Apparently, the development of subjective sleepiness is similar across night driving studies. It should be pointed out that the time on task effect in night driving studies will contain effects of increased time awake and effects of the circadian downswing of alertness. However, Sagaspe and colleagues[30] actually controlled for these factors by measuring sleepiness (KSS) at 5 a.m. after 8 hours, 4 hours, or 2 hours of driving during the night (and normal sleep duration the night before). The effect was a significant increase of ≈KSS = 1 across these durations. Zero hours of duration was unfortunately not used in this study, but the results show that there is an increase in time on task effects even beyond that occurring after 2 hours.

Taken together, sleepiness is increased to high levels during night driving and during morning driving after a night spent awake. Also, driving behavior is impaired, even if there is a lack of sleepiness measures immediately preceding road crashes.

EARLY MORNING WORK

Morning work has seldom been investigated in terms of sleepiness or accidents despite the fact that they interfere with sleep. One of the few studies of sleepiness after early starts (at 5 or 6 a.m.) measured sleepiness among bus drivers in the afternoon (in a split shift system with no work during the middle of the day).[31] EEG sleep indicators and blink durations and sleepiness (KSS, mean = 5.8, compared with 3.4 after no work in the morning) increased after an early morning start. Similar results have been demonstrated for train drivers[32] and cabin crew.[33] Both studies showed correlation with sleep duration. Studies of the morning shift in traditional industrial shift work also show increased sleepiness during the rest of the day.[34]

The reason for sleepiness in morning work is, logically, the shortening of sleep duration with earlier shift start times.[35] It seems that for each hour of phase advance, sleep duration decreases by 40 to 50 minutes.[36] The latter study was representative of the Swedish population and therefore represents industry and health care, as well as transport. It also seems the case that sleep is not only shorter in morning work, but also contains less of sleep stage N3 (deep sleep), particularly if the early rising is anticipated with apprehension.[33]

THE IMPERATIVE POWER OF SLEEPINESS

Previously, it was concluded that EEG and EOG measures show that incursions of sleep during work/activity, and accidents occur during while driving at night on real roads with normal traffic density. Comparisons with alcohol effects indicate that late night sleepiness causes behavioral impairment similar to that of 0.05% to 0.08% blood alcohol levels.[37,38] This suggests that sleepiness is a powerful force. But, how imperative is it?

One glimpse of the imperative nature of sleepiness comes from a driving simulator study of the effects of rumble strips.[39] It was found that hitting a rumble strip in the morning after being awake during the night was associated with strong prehit increases in EEG alpha/theta activity, eye closure duration, lateral variability of the vehicle, and high sleepiness levels (KSS = 8.1 on the 9-step scale). Thus, sleepiness was undoubtedly present for at least 5 minutes before hitting the rumble strip, and no further increase was seen immediately before the hit. The hit immediately reduced EOG, EEG, and driving variability to intermediate levels of sleepiness and the vehicle was brought back to the proper lane by the driver. But, the increased alertness was reversed in 2 to 4 minutes, and a new hit occurred some minutes later. This was repeated 7 more times on the average and with gradually decreasing intervals.[40] Apparently, the alerting effects of a hit were extremely temporary,

and irresistible sleepiness returned very rapidly, despite major efforts to remain awake. Despite the loud noise from the rumble strip, the tilt of the vehicle, and the abrupt awakening, most participants continued to fall asleep. Sleepiness seems imperative.

AWARENESS OF SLEEPINESS

Apparently, individuals are aware of their sleepy state, as subjective ratings of sleepiness are increased before a real road accident[5] and before driving off the road in a driving simulator.[41,42] This suggests that the afflicted person either fails to realize that his or her state is dangerous or that sleepiness, while perceived as high, still seems possible to handle. There remains, however, an attempt to turn off consciousness by the brain without a final warning, somewhat like the state instability characterizing states of sleep loss.[43,44] The instability occurs at relatively high levels of sleep loss (24 hours awake), and involves short, relatively frequent reductions of prefrontal cortex metabolism, combined with high levels that seem related to efforts to fight sleepiness. The decision not to stop driving or employ effective countermeasures may be related to a high degree of confidence in one's own ability to resist sleepiness, perhaps based previous success in similar situations. Probably also the reluctance to delay the time reach the endpoint of the trip contributes to decisions not to stop.

SLEEP

Impaired sleep is part of the problem of sleepy driving, but has rather seldom been investigated. Sleep has mainly been studied in traditional industrial shift work. Other studies include those from Sallinen and Kecklund,[45] Linton and colleagues,[46] and Kecklund and Axelsson.[47] Obviously, night shift work that covers the period between 10 p.m. and 6 a.m. does not contain any sleep, except perhaps a nap. However, transport work can end and start at many different times of day. **Fig. 2** depicts sleep duration after different bed times for French train drivers, actually the first study to use polysomnography to record sleep in shift workers.[48] The figure shows how sleep becomes shorter the later sleep starts (after the drivers have worked part of the night). Toward noon, sleep duration seems to start rising again. This dependence of sleep on the bedtime after work has been demonstrated repeatedly.

The results of Foret and colleagues were confirmed in a study of truck drivers interviewed

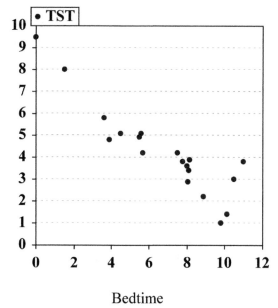

Fig. 2. Sleep duration after different bed times for French train drivers.

at rest stops on French motorways. The results showed that sleep duration became shorter with increasing earliness of rising, and with increasing earliness of start time of the drive.[49] Overall, 12.7% of the drivers had slept less than 6 hours on the night before the interview.

The only PSG study of sleep in truck drivers (long-haul (10 or 13-hour drives)) showed less than 4 hours (mean across a work week) for a steady night schedule, and less than 5 hours for both gradually advancing and delaying nigh drive schedules.[19] Even steady day driving was associated with only 5.4 hours of sleep. Naps added an average of 0.45 hours. Pylkkönen and colleagues[21] followed a group of long-haul truck drivers across 2 weeks, with actigraphy. Morning shifts were preceded by 5:43 hours of sleep and day shifts by at least 7 hours. The amounts of sleep are low in both studies.

The sleep duration in the studies of truck drivers described previously are surprisingly short. In studies of industrial shift workers, the amounts are rather similar. The sleep after a night shift is usually initiated 1 hour after the termination of the shift[50,51] with little variation (30–60 min standard deviation) between individuals. The ensuing sleep is, according to EEG-studies, reduced by 2 to 4 hours.[34] Most of the loss involves stage 2 and rapid eye movement (REM) sleep, whereas slow-wave sleep (SWS) is unaffected. The subjective aspects of sleep seem little affected, apart from the reports of premature awakenings, and of not getting enough sleep.[52] Interestingly, about

50% experience a spontaneous (and effortless) sleep termination.[52] About one-third of the shift workers add a late afternoon nap between the subsequent night shifts.[50,51] The nap duration often exceeds 1 hour, and the prevalence of napping increases with decreasing length of the prior main sleep.[53,54] Thus, the nap seems to be a compensation for insufficient prior sleep.

A morning shift in industrial shift work usually spans the time between 6 a.m. and 2 p.m., but variations occur, particularly so in transport. The sleep pattern appears even more rigid in connection with the morning shift than in connection with the night shift.[55] The short sleep (6 hours) has also been demonstrated in EEG studies; usually a 2- to 4-hour reduction of sleep length occurs.[56] Again, mainly stage 2 and REM are affected. The main subjective effect is pronounced difficulties awakening, nonspontaneous awakening, and a feeling of not being refreshed by sleep.[52] The difficulties awakening often make the morning shift the most disliked of the 3 shifts. Again, however, the quality of sleep, in itself, does not seem to be affected. Interestingly, the anticipation of difficulties awakening is associated with reduced SWS.[33] Thus, sleep before the morning shift seems to contain an extra dimension of sleep disturbance, apart from reduced length.

THE MECHANISM

In the introduction it was briefly mentioned that shift work is a problem when it interferes with normal sleep hours. A night shift displaces work to the window of circadian low, when metabolism is slow, and sleepiness/fatigue is induced.[57,58] Because the night worker usually will spend daytime before shift start awake, the number of hours will increase to approximately 22 hours (14 hours awake before first night shift starts) when the morning shift ends, as compared with 10 hours (2 hours awake before shift start) before a morning shift ends. The number of hours spent awake will gradually increase sleepiness.[58,59] The amount of prior sleep before a night shift is usually quite normal, or even a bit increased if the worker is trying to bank sleep before the first night shift. If the night shift is preceded by another night shift, prior sleep will have taken place between 7 or 8 a.m., and 1 or 2 p.m., probably somewhat shortened. The combined effects of time of day, time awake, and sleep loss have been turned into mathematical models, and the first published model was that of Folkard and Åkerstedt,[60] which has subsequently been updated many times.

SHIFT WORK DISORDER AND COUNTERMEASURES

There are individual differences in the ability to tolerate shift work. Older age, morning-type personality, and high need for sleep have been suggested, but seem to explain little of interindividual differences in vulnerability.[61–63] In another approach, Axelsson and colleagues[64] compared shift workers who were negative to shift work with those who were neutral or positive. Several predictors were tested (eg, age, gender, and sleep need), and the most important one was high sleepiness during night shifts among the negative shift workers. Sleep duration in relation to night shifts did not differ.

Similar vulnerability is the basis of the diagnosis shift work disorder (SWD). This has been formalized in the diagnosis SWD, which has been the focus of at least 2 previous articles in this journal[61,62] and in another journal.[63] Briefly, it describes insomnia and/or excessive sleepiness occurring during work hours that interfere with the normal work hours (but not during day-oriented living). There is no clear operational definition of the condition; it is mainly a question of severity of the symptoms. The prevalence is estimated to 5% to 10% of shift workers.[62] No data are available on the prevalence in the transport sector specifically. It is also not known if shift work actually causes SWD or if certain individuals from the start are less able to sleep after a night shift or less able to maintain adequate alertness during night shifts. However, entering shift work is associated with increased sleep/alertness problems, but these seem to recede on leaving shift work.[65]

Among countermeasures, bright light treatment during night work seems successful,[66] but not feasible in truck drivers during the night. In 1 study, blue light increased alertness during night driving.[67] Naps and caffeine have been repeatedly investigated as alertness-promoting factors in connection with night work.[68] Also alertness-enhancing drugs like armodafinil improve night driving performance, but some fatigue effects remain.[69] Melatonin has frequently been suggested as a means to promote day sleep after a night shift.[70] No countermeasure seems to have reached widespread use.

With respect to treatment, cognitive behavioral therapy for insomnia (CBT-I) appears to partially improve sleep in shift workers.[71] In a different approach with 53 Finnish truck drivers, an alertness training program gave advice on sleep and alertness regulation, including countermeasures in a subgroup.[72] The change in sleepiness (KSS) from 2 weeks before to 2 weeks after the program was not significant, however. Apparently there is need for more treatment interventions in SWD.

SUMMARY

Driving a vehicle during a night shift increases the accident risk and incidents of falling asleep at the wheel. Individuals having worked a night shift (in any type of occupation) run a similar risk when commuting home from a night shift. Early starts of driving may increase risk. Detailed field studies of sleepiness indicate high levels of sleepiness during late night driving. The mechanism includes exposure to the circadian trough of alertness during work and sleep loss. High levels of sleepiness and sleep loss associated with night and early morning work define the diagnosis of SWD. Interventions or treatments to mitigate sleep and fatigue problems in shift work are rarely implemented.

Shift work that includes night shifts causes high levels of sleepiness that may constitute a major safety risk, particularly in transport work, but also in health care and industry. The reason is a misalignment between the night-oriented work/rest pattern and the day-oriented circadian system. The impact of sleepiness is powerful, and lapses of consciousness may occur at high levels of sleepiness without any additional warning. Particularly vulnerable subjects, around 8% to 10%, are at a special risk and may be diagnosed with SWD. This group also suffers from increased sleepiness during other shifts and spends much of its waking hours at pathologic sleepiness levels. Countermeasures/treatments include naps, improved sleep schedules, light treatment, alertness-enhancing drugs, rapid shift rotation, and clockwise shift rotation.

REFERENCES

1. Bioulac S, Micoulaud-Franchi JA, Arnaud M, et al. Risk of motor vehicle accidents related to sleepiness at the wheel: a systematic review and meta-analysis. Sleep 2017;40(10):1–10.
2. Higgins JS, Michael J, Austin R, et al. Asleep at the wheel-the road to addressing drowsy driving. Sleep 2017;40(2):1–9.
3. Stutts JC, Wilkins JW, Vaughn BV. Why do people have drowsy driving crashes? Input from drivers who just dit. Washington, DC: AAA Foundation for Traffic Safety; 1999. 202/638-5944.
4. McCartt AT, Ribner SA, Pack AI, et al. The scope and nature of the drowsy driving problem in New York State. Accid Anal Prev 1996;28(4):511–7.

5. Connor J, Norton R, Ameratunga S, et al. Driver sleepiness and risk of serious injury to car occupants: population based case control study. BMJ 2002;324(7346):1125.

6. Crummy F, Cameron PA, Swann P, et al. Prevalence of sleepiness in surviving drivers of motor vehicle collisions. Intern Med J 2008;38(10):769–75.

7. Hakkanen H, Summala H. Sleepiness at work among commercial truck drivers. Sleep 2000;23(1): 49–57.

8. Marcus CL, Loughlin GM. Effect of sleep deprivation on driving safety in housestaff. Sleep 1996;19(10): 763–6.

9. Gold DR, Rogacz S, Bock N, et al. Rotating shift work, sleep, and accidents related to sleepiness in hospital nurses. Am J Public Health 1992;82(7): 1011–4.

10. Barger LK, Cade BE, Ayas NT, et al. Extended work shifts and the risk of motor vehicle crashes among interns. N Engl J Med 2005;352:125–34.

11. Scott LD, Hwang WT, Rogers AE, et al. The relationship between nurse work schedules, sleep duration, and drowsy driving. Sleep 2007;30(12):1801–7.

12. Harris W. Fatigue, circadian rhythm and truck accidents. In: Mackie RR, editor. Vigilance. New York: Plenum Press; 1977. p. 133–46.

13. Hamelin P. Lorry driver's time habits in work and their involvement in traffic accidents. Ergonomics 1987; 30:1323–33.

14. Langlois PH, Smolensky MH, Hsi BP, et al. Temporal patterns of reported single-vehicle car and truck accidents in Texas, USA during 1980-1983. Chronobiol Int 1985;2(2):131–46.

15. Åkerstedt T, Kecklund G, Hörte L-G. Night driving, season, and the risk of highway accidents. Sleep 2001;24:401–6.

16. Åkerstedt T, Kecklund G. Age, gender and early morning highway accidents. J Sleep Res 2001;10: 105–10.

17. Hanowski RJ, Wierwille WW, Dingus TA. An on-road study to investigate fatigue in local/short haul trucking. Accid Anal Prev 2003;35(2):153–60.

18. Klauer SG, Dingus TA, Neale VL, et al. The impact of driver inattention on near-crash/cash-risk: an analysis using the 100-car naturalistic driving study data. Blacksburg (VA):: Virginia Tech Transportation Institute; 2006.

19. Mitler MM, Miller JC, Lipsitz JJ, et al. The sleep of long-haul truck drivers. N Engl J Med 1997;337: 755–61.

20. Kecklund G, Åkerstedt T. Sleepiness in long distance truck driving: an ambulatory EEG study of night driving. Ergonomics 1993;36(9):1007–17.

21. Pylkkonen M, Sihvola M, Hyvarinen HK, et al. Sleepiness, sleep, and use of sleepiness countermeasures in shift-working long-haul truck drivers. Accid Anal Prev 2015;80:201–10.

22. Åkerstedt T, Gillberg M. Subjective and objective sleepiness in the active individual. Int J Neurosci 1990;52:29–37.

23. Torsvall L, Åkerstedt T. Sleepiness during day and night work: a field study of train drivers. Sleep Res 1983;12:376.

24. Åkerstedt T, Hallvig D, Anund A, et al. Having to stop driving at night because of dangerous sleepiness - awareness, physiology and behaviour. J Sleep Res 2013;22(4):380–8.

25. Hallvig D, Anund A, Fors C, et al. Real driving at night - predicting lane departures from physiological and subjective sleepiness. Biol Psychol 2014;101: 18–23.

26. Sandberg D, Anund A, Fors C, et al. The characteristics of sleepiness during real driving at night–a study of driving performance, physiology and subjective experience. Sleep 2011;34(10): 1317–25.

27. Anderson C, Ftouni S, Ronda JM, et al. Self-reported drowsiness and safety outcomes while driving after an extended duration work shift in trainee physicians. Sleep 2018;41(2):1–12.

28. Lee ML, Howard ME, Horrey WJ, et al. High risk of near-crash driving events following night-shift work. Proc Natl Acad Sci U S A 2016;113(1):176–81.

29. Perrier J, Jongen S, Vuurman E, et al. Driving performance and EEG fluctuations during on-the-road driving following sleep deprivation. Biol Psychol 2016;121(Pt A):1–11.

30. Sagaspe P, Taillard J, Akerstedt T, et al. Extended driving impairs nocturnal driving performances. PLoS One 2008;3(10):e3493.

31. Anund A, Fors C, Ihlstrom J, et al. An on-road study of sleepiness in split shifts among city bus drivers. Accid Anal Prev 2018;114:71–6.

32. Ingre M, Kecklund G, Åkerstedt T, et al. Variation in sleepiness during early morning shifts: a mixed model approach to an experimental field study of train drivers. Chronobiol Int 2004;21:973–90.

33. Kecklund G, Åkerstedt T, Lowden A. Morning work: effects of early rising on sleep and alertness. Sleep 1997;20(3):215–23.

34. Kecklund G, Åkerstedt T. Effects of timing of shifts on sleepiness and sleep duration. J Sleep Res 1995;4(S2):47–50.

35. Ingre M, Kecklund G, Akerstedt T, et al. Sleep length as a function of morning shift-start time in irregular shift schedules for train drivers: self-rated health and individual differences. Chronobiol Int 2008; 25(2):349–58.

36. Akerstedt T, Kecklund G, Selén J. Early morning work - prevalence and relation to sleep/wake problems: a national representative survey. Chronobiol Int 2010;27(5):975–86.

37. Dawson D, Reid K. Fatigue, alcohol and performance impairment. Nature 1997;388:235.

38. Arnedt JT, Owens J, Crouch M, et al. Neurobehavioral performance of residents after heavy night call vs after alcohol ingestion. JAMA 2005;294(9):1025–33.

39. Anund A, Kecklund G, Vadeby A, et al. The alerting effect of hitting a rumble strip-A simulator study with sleepy drivers. Accid Anal Prev 2008;40(6):1970–6.

40. Watling CN, Akerstedt T, Kecklund G, et al. Do repeated rumble strip hits improve driver alertness? J Sleep Res 2016;25(2):241–7.

41. Horne JA, Baulk SD. Awareness of sleepiness when driving. Psychophysiology 2004;41:161–5.

42. Ingre M, Akerstedt T, Peters B, et al. Subjective sleepiness and accident risk avoiding the ecological fallacy. J Sleep Res 2006;15(2):142–8.

43. Van Dongen HPA, Vitellaro KM, Dinges DF. Individual differences in adult human sleep and wakefulness: leitmotif for a research agenda. Sleep 2005;28:479–96.

44. Lim J, Dinges DF. A meta-analysis of the impact of short-term sleep deprivation on cognitive variables. Psychol Bull 2010;136(3):375–89.

45. Sallinen M, Kecklund G. Shift work, sleep and sleepiness - differences between shift schedules and systems. Scand J Work Environ Health 2010;36(2):121–33.

46. Linton SJ, Kecklund G, Franklin KA, et al. The effect of the work environment on future sleep disturbances: a systematic review. Sleep Med Rev 2015;23:10–9.

47. Kecklund G, Axelsson J. Health consequences of shift work and insufficient sleep. BMJ 2016;355:i5210.

48. Foret J, Lantin G. The sleep of train drivers: an example of the effects of irregular work schedules on sleep. In: Colquhoun WP, editor. Aspects of human efficiency. Diurnal rhythm and loss of sleep. London: The English Universities Press Ltd; 1972. p. 273–81.

49. Philip P, Taillard J, Léger D, et al. Work and rest sleep schedules of 227 European truck drivers. Sleep Med 2002;3:507–11.

50. Knauth P, Rutenfranz J. Duration of sleep related to the type of shift work. In: Reinberg A, Vieux N, Andlauer P, editors. Night and shift work: biological and social aspects. Oxford (United Kingdom): Pergamon Press; 1981.

51. Tepas DI. Shiftworker sleep strategies. J Hum Ergol (Tokyo) 1982;11(Suppl):325–36.

52. Åkerstedt T, Kecklund G, Knutsson A. Spectral analysis of sleep electroencephalography in rotating three-shift work. Scand J Work Environ Health 1991;17:330–6.

53. Rosa R. Napping at home and alertness on the job in rotating shift workers. Sleep 1993;16(8):727–35.

54. Åkerstedt T, Torsvall L. Napping in shift work. Sleep 1985;8(2):105–9.

55. Folkard S, Barton J. Does the "forbidden zone" for sleep onset influence morning shift sleep duration? Ergonomics 1993;36(1–3):85–91.

56. Åkerstedt T. Work hours, sleepiness and accidents introduction and summary. J Sleep Res 1995;4(suppl 2):1–3.

57. Folkard S, Åkerstedt T. A three process model of the regulation of alertness and sleepiness. In: Ogilvie R, Broughton R, editors. Sleep, arousal and performance: problems and promises. Boston: Birkhäuser; 1991. p. 11–26.

58. Dijk D-J, Czeisler CA. Contribution of the circadian pacemaker and the sleep homeostat to sleep propensity, sleep structure, electroencephalographic slow waves, and sleep spindle activity in humans. J Neurosci 1995;15(5):3526–38.

59. Fröberg JE. Twenty-four hour patterns in human performance, subjective and physiological variables and differences between morning and evening active subjects. Biol Psychol 1977;5:119–34.

60. Folkard S, Åkerstedt T. Towards a model for the prediction of alertness and/or fatigue on different sleep/wake schedules. In: Oginski A, Pokorski J, Rutenfranz J, editors. Contemporary advances in shiftwork research. Krakow (Poland): Medical Academy; 1987. p. 231–40.

61. Akerstedt T, Wright KP. Sleep loss and fatigue in shift work and shift work disorder. Sleep Med Clin 2009;4(2):257–71.

62. Reid KJ, Abbott SM. Jet lag and shift work disorder. Sleep Med Clin 2015;10(4):523–35.

63. Wickwire EM, Geiger-Brown J, Scharf SM, et al. Shift work and shift work sleep disorder: clinical and organizational perspectives. Chest 2017;151(5):1156–72.

64. Axelsson J, Åkerstedt T, Kecklund G, et al. Tolerance to shift work - how does it relate to sleep and wakefullness? Int Arch Occup Environ Health 2004;77:121–9.

65. Akerstedt T, Nordin M, Alfredsson L, et al. Sleep and sleepiness: impact of entering or leaving shiftwork - a prospective study. Chronobiol Int 2010;27(5):987–96.

66. Dawson D, Encel N, Lushington K. Improving adaptation to simulated night shift: timed exposure to bright light versus daytime melatonin administration. Sleep 1995;18:11–21.

67. Taillard J, Capelli A, Sagaspe P, et al. In-car nocturnal blue light exposure improves motorway driving: a randomized controlled trial. PLoS One 2012;7(10):e46750.

68. Schweitzer PK, Randazzo AC, Stone K, et al. Laboratory and field studies of naps and caffeine as practical countermeasures for sleep-wake problems associated with night work. Sleep 2006;29(1):39–50.

69. Drake C, Gumenyuk V, Roth T, et al. Effects of armodafinil on simulated driving and alertness in shift work disorder. Sleep 2014;37(12):1987–94.

70. Smith MR, Lee C, Crowley SJ, et al. Morning melatonin has limited benefit as a soporific for daytime sleep after night work. Chronobiol Int 2005;22(5): 873–88.

71. Järnefelt H, Lagerstedt R, Kajaste S, et al. Cognitive behavioral therapy for shift workers with chronic insomnia. Sleep Med 2012;13(10):1238–46.

72. Pylkkonen M, Tolvanen A, Hublin C, et al. Effects of alertness management training on sleepiness among long-haul truck drivers: a randomized controlled trial. Accid Anal Prev 2018;121:301–13.

The Economic Burden of Sleepy Driving

Damien Léger, MD, PhD[a,b,*], Emilie Pepin, MD[a,b], Gabriela Caetano, MD[b]

KEYWORDS

- Driving sleepy • Motor vehicle accident • Costs • Productivity • Occupational accidents–economy

KEY POINTS

- The economic burden of sleepy driving includes direct costs of accidents and indirect costs of lost lives, disability, lost productivity, and occupational and civil accidents.
- Sleepy driving is mainly due to sleep restriction associated with work schedules or poor sleep hygiene. Sleep disorders, like obstructive sleep apnea (OSA) and central hypersomnia, and treatment with sedative drugs, however, also have to be screened.
- The authors hypothesize that the costs of accidents due to sleepiness could be in the United States between $139 billion and $152 billion and in Europe between €43 billion and €337 billion.
- Based on 1.3 million sleepy drivers dying on the world's roads every year, including 400,000 under age 25 years and 400,000 above age 65 years, it may be estimated that the indirect cost of sleepy driving on society is $2372 billion per year.
- Based on the 20 million to 50 million sleepy drivers who are injured or disabled, the cost of disability for insurance may be hypothesized to be between $2580 billion and $6450 billion every year.

INTRODUCTION

Driving while sleepy is now widely recognized by health authorities and by general opinion as a major behavioral risk of accidents. Several major public campaigns have been launched on that timely topic in the United States, in Europe, in Australia, and in other parts of the world.[1–5] Public health messages have been extensively given by experts urging drivers to stop for a nap or a break every 2 hours on long trips, to avoid driving at night, and to sleep adequately in a 24-hour cycle. Drivers have been also informed to see their doctors when they have had near-miss accidents or sleepiness at the wheel on a regular basis to investigate and treat potential sleep disorders, such as obstructive sleep apnea (OSA) or central hypersomnia.

The main causes of driving while sleepy may be divided in 2 categories:

- The first and by far the most frequent cause of sleepiness at the wheel is a behavioral one. In most of the industrialized countries, 20% to 35% of adults are sleeping less than 6 hours per 24 hours[6–8] and, therefore, are sleepy during daytime, with a higher risk of sleepy driving. This sleep debt has several determinants, which are
  - Night work and shift work, which are consensually recognized as having an

Disclosure Statement: Dr D. Léger is or has been consulted as the main investigator in studies sponsored by Actelion, Agence Spatiale Européenne, Ag2R, Bioprojet, CNES (France), DGA, iSommeil, Jazz, Jannsen, Vanda (United States), Merck (United States), NASA (United States), Philips (United States), ResMed, Sanofi (France), Rhythm, Vinci Foundation, and VitalAire in the past 5 years. He declares no conflict of interest in relation to this article. E. Pepin and G. Caetano have no disclosures to report.
[a] Université de Paris, Paris Descartes, EA 7330 VIFASOM (Vigilance Fatigue Sommeil et santé Publique), 15 rue de l'Ecole de Médecine, Paris 75006, France; [b] Assistance Publique Hôpitaux de Paris, APHP-5, Hôtel-Dieu de Paris, Centre du Sommeil et de la Vigilance, 1 place du Parvis Notre-Dame, Paris 75181 PARIS CEDEX 04, France
* Corresponding author. Université Paris Descartes, Hôtel-Dieu APHP, Centre du Sommeil et de la Vigilance, 1 place du Parvis Notre-Dame, Paris 75181 PARIS CEDEX 04, France.
E-mail address: damien.leger@aphp.fr

Sleep Med Clin 14 (2019) 423–429
https://doi.org/10.1016/j.jsmc.2019.07.004
1556-407X/19/© 2019 Elsevier Inc. All rights reserved.

impact on sleep length, with an average reduction of 1 hour per 24 hours compared with the sleep time of day workers[9–11]

  ○ Connection time between work and home, which increases continuously among big towns and in nonindustrialized countries, with workers arriving later and later at home and departing earlier and earlier in the morning, increasing periods of wakefulness in 24 hours and having an impact on sleepiness at the wheel[12–14]

  ○ Leisure and overuse of screens, smartphones, and videogames later and later in the evening and even at night, disrupting and reducing sleep not only of teens and young adults but also of more and more older adults[15–17]

- The second cause is associated with sleep disorders, which are well described in this issue, specifically OSA; insomnia treated with some kind of long-term sedative treatments; and rare forms of central hypersomnia, such as narcolepsy. All these sleep disorders have been extensively associated with an increased risk of accidents.[18–20]

Whatever the causes of driving sleepy, the burden is similar and may be divided as

- Direct costs of driving while sleepy, which include the human and material costs of motor vehicle accidents (MVAs) (while at work and while driving for leisure), including material loss and hospitalizations and health care directly associated with being sleepy

- Indirect costs of absenteeism, loss of productivity, loss of opportunity, loss of education, loss of income, and impaired quality of life

THE DIRECT COSTS OF SLEEPY DRIVING
Magnitude of Motor Vehicle Accidents

Globally around the world, MVAs are the third most common cause of death. They affect young adults, specifically, however, for whom they are the first cause. Car accidents claim approximately 1.3 million lives every year, according to the Association for Safe International Road Travel.[21] Twenty million to 50 million people are injured or disabled each year as well. More than half of all road traffic deaths occur among young adults. Road crashes are the leading cause of death worldwide among young people and the second leading cause of death among those between 5 to 14 years old. Each year, approximately 400,000 people under 25 die on the world's roads, on average of more than 1000 a day. In the United States alone, road crashes account for more than 37,000 of those fatalities and 2.35 million injuries.[21]

The Direct Costs of Accidents

In the United States alone, a 2014 National Highway Traffic Safety Administration (NHTSA) study showed that MVAs had an $871 billion economic and societal impact on US citizens.[22] This report also shows that in 2013, there were more than 32,000 crash deaths in the United States. These deaths cost more than $380 million in direct medical costs.

In Europe, a recent review estimates the costs of injuries and fatalities due to MVAs per country in relation to the gross domestic product (GDP).[23] Reported costs per fatality vary between €0.7 million per fatality in Slovakia and €3.0 million per fatality in Austria and tend to be higher in Northwest Europe than in South and East Europe. Reported costs per serious injury range from €28,000 in Latvia to €959,000 in Estonia, whereas reported costs per slight injury range from €296 in Latvia to €71,742 in Iceland. When the costs per injury are related to the costs per fatality, they show that the costs of a serious injury range from 2.5% to 34% of the costs of a fatality, although for approximately three-quarters of the countries this figure is between 10% and 20%. The costs per slight injury were 0.03% to 4.2% of the costs of a fatality. The total costs of crashes vary between 0.4% and 4.1% of the GDP.[23]

Differences between countries throughout Europe are also due to methodology, particularly whether the willingness to pay (WTP) method is applied for the calculation of human costs. In countries that use the WTP approach, human costs have a major share (34% to 91%) in the total costs of crashes. In countries that apply an alternative method, the share of human costs in the total costs is much smaller (less than 10%). The standard costs of a fatality are estimated at €2.3 million. These costs mainly consist of human cost (€1.6 million) and production loss (€0.7 million). Costs per serious and slight injury are estimated at 13% and 1% of the value of a fatality. Also, for injuries, human costs are by far the largest cost item. Total costs according to the international guidelines in all European Union (EU) countries individually as well as the EU in total were calculated. For the 28 EU member states, costs are estimated at approximately €270 billion if the results of the value transfer approach are applied. This corresponds to 1.8% of GDP.[23]

The Direct Costs of Accidents Due to Sleepiness

It has been postulated that sleepiness causes 16% of all road MVAs and more than 20% of motorway crashes[24] and that between 30% and 50% of deaths and serious injuries in accidents are caused by sleep-related Road traffic accidents.[25] Based on the previous estimate of the costs of accidents, it may, therefore, be hypothesized that the costs of accidents due to sleepiness in the United States could be between $139.4 billion (16% of $871 billion) and $152 billion (0.4 (between 30% and 50%) × 380 billion).

In Europe, these costs are estimated between €43 billion (16% of €270 billion) and €337 billion (gross national product of Europe €18.774 billion × 1.8%).

The US NHTSA estimates that drowsy driving was responsible for 72,000 crashes, 44,000 injuries, and 800 deaths in 2013. These numbers are underestimated, however, and up to 6000 fatal crashes each year may be caused by drowsy drivers.[26] In 2016, according to the NHTSA, drowsy drivers cost society an estimated $109 billion per year.

In Australia, the cost to the community of drowsy driving road accidents is estimated to be $2 billion every year with MVAs, which may be divided into $530 million due to excessive daytime sleepiness (EDS) related to sleep deprivation, $862 million due to other causes of EDS, and $740 million due to insufficient sleep.[27]

In Brazil, in 2004, there were 97,074 deaths per day and 4.072 deaths per hour, or 1.018 deaths every 15 minutes, resulting from traffic accidents, with a total financial cost of $28.95 billion. Based on sleepiness-attributed accidents rates in Brazil, 17.60 deaths per day or 0.73 deaths per hour are associated with sleepy driving, with a total financial cost of $414,397,997 as a consequence of traffic-related deaths in 2004, a major cause of which was sleepy driving.[28]

The Direct Costs of Accidents Due to Sleepiness in Obstructive Sleep Apnea Patients

There is limited literature trying to assess the cost of EDS or driving sleepy in addition to the other direct or indirect costs of OSA. A Frost & Sullivan report, however, ordered by the American Academy of Sleep Medicine (AASM) in the United States, *Hidden Health Crisis Costing America Billions*, suggests some possible answers.[29] The report estimates that approximatively $12.4 billion was spent in the United States in 2015 diagnosing and treating OSA for the 5.9 million US adults

diagnosed with the disease, a larger and more significant investment of approximatively $49.5 billion would be necessary for the 23.5 million individuals with OSA who were undiagnosed at this time. The report compared this direct cost to the indirect ones that result from not being treated. They specifically estimated that the indirect cost of nontreated OSA was $26.2 billion for MVAs, $6.5 billion for workplace accidents, and $86.9 billion per year for lost productivity.[29] Another Frost & Sullivan report ordered by the AASM focused on treated OSA patients. It postulated that treatment induced a 40% decline in workplaces absences and a 17.3% increase in productivity.[30] Thus, treatment would potentially be able to cost-save most of the sleepiness consequences of driving sleepy in OSA patients. It cannot be concluded, however, that all the costs associated to sleepiness at the job in OSA patients are specifically linked to diving sleepy. Only one proportion is responsible, which cannot be exactly calculated.

THE INDIRECT COSTS OF ACCIDENTS DUE TO SLEEPINESS
The "Value" of Human Life

Apart from the direct costs of accidents, the worst impact on society due to accidents is the loss of human beings potentially involved in the future economic network of their countries. One human life is priceless. Aside from the methodology of WTP, described previously, insurance companies and public authorities also traditionally base their estimates on the price of 1 human life after an accident. It is estimated by the total income a person would have earned in a total lifetime until age 60s. Then, when a person under 25 dies on the road, this means 35 years of income is lost. The individual yearly income varies extensively from one country to another depending on the national gross product income of each country and each socioprofessional category. In the United States, the average lifetime earnings for college graduates was estimated to be $2.4 million in 2017.[31] In Europe, the standard costs of a fatality for an adult is €2.3 million.[32] After age 65, the insurance companies usually apply a senior discount rate, which takes more account of the moral impact of death on those nearest than of the economic impact. For household people in the United States, the average compensation was estimated to be $80,000.[32]

The Indirect Costs of Sleepy Driving on Lost Human Lives

Part of the 1.3 million are dying including 400000 under 25 age and 400000 above 65 age, it may be estimated, based on Western values of life, that the indirect costs of sleepy driving to society are $(600,000 \times 2.3 + 400,000 \times 2.4 + 400,000 \times 0.08) = \$2372$ billion.

The Indirect Costs of Sleepy Driving on Disability

In Western developed countries, another method of assessing human cost values is to estimate how much insurance companies must pay to give 1 year of quality life to disabled or injured people. For a long time, it has been estimated at $50,000 or less. New research, however, has proposed that in the United States, that figure was far too low. Recently, Princeton University economists have demonstrated that the average value of a year of quality human life was actually closer to approximately $129,000 per year.[33] Based on the 20 million to 50 million people who are injured or disabled, the cost of disability for insurance may be hypothesized at $2580 billion to $6450 billion every year.

The Indirect Costs of Driving While Sleepy on the Loss of Productivity

Driving while sleepy may affect productivity in different ways besides the one of Motor vehicle accidents at work, discussed previously.

- First, it may be hypothesized that a sleepy driver drives more slowly and makes mistakes on the itinerary, which may have consequences on the delivery of goods by the driver. It is difficult to accurately assess how this delay may affect productivity. Delays caused by late shipments, however, can slow down an assembly line's productivity. Inevitably money is lost because employees who are not working at their top speed and efficiency cost money. The production time is longer, because additional time is spent waiting for shipments, all the while having employees on the clock for hours or days longer than they should be. What is more, there are higher inventory costs because of these delays. There is a timeline and a budget for each good production project, and there should be confidence in the ability to accomplish them quickly and in a streamlined fashion. If engaged with a dependable supplier, these additional costs created by low productivity can be avoided.
- Moreover, if a customer's orders are delayed due to late shipments from suppliers, souring important relationships and ultimately decreasing customer satisfaction

are risked. If clients are continuously forced to wait for their orders due to late shipments, they might take their business to competitors. Losing customers means losing out on money, which critically affects the bottom line.

The authors did not find any literature on the cost of sleepy driving on productivity. They did find, however, recent works on driving while sleepy at work, which may help in understanding the magnitude of this burden. A survey of 2189 truck drivers was recently made by researchers of the Safety and Health Assessment and Research for Prevention program, of Washington State, enquiring about the perception of associated with work-related injury. Daytime sleepiness, pressure to work faster, driving less than truckload, and having a poor composite score for safety perceptions all were associated with increased likelihood of work-related injury.[34]

In Australia, Bruck[27] also estimated the cost of loss productivity not only due to driving sleepy but also due to injuries promoted by EDS. Based on the results of Safe Work Australia (2015) and the average annual earnings in Australia in 2013, it was estimated that the productivity has an impact on per workplace injury due to EDS-sleep debt would be equivalent to 1.22 times the average annual earnings of the general population. This was estimated to cost Australian $1 billion in 2016 to 2017. In another recent Australian national survey, the aim was also to test the relationship between sleep duration and disorders, sleep health and hygiene factors, and work-related factors and errors at work in Australian workers. A group of 512 workers provided responses to the question, "Thinking about the past 3 months, how many days did you make errors at work because you were too sleepy or you had a sleep problem?"[35] Work errors related to sleepiness or sleep problems were found 11.6 times higher ($P<.001$) in those who snored, 7.0 times higher in short ($\leq$5 h/night) sleepers ($P<.021$), and 6.1 times higher in those staying up later than planned most nights of the week ($P<.001$). It may, therefore, be hypothesized that sleepy drivers may also have an impact on safety and productivity in the workplace through increased sleepiness-related errors.

Finally, Redeker and colleagues[36] also recently analyzed 60 articles on workplace interventions made to promote sleep health and an alert, healthy workforce. They suggest that employer-sponsored efforts can improve sleep and sleep-related outcomes at the workplace. They conclude that employers encouraging better sleep habits and general fitness results in self-reported improvements in sleep-related outcomes and may be associated with reduced absenteeism and better overall quality of life.[36]

THE BURDEN OF SLEEPY DRIVING IN THE RISK OF OCCUPATIONAL AND PUBLIC ACCIDENTS
Occupational Accidents

There are few data specifically devoted to the cost of occupational accidents associated with driving while sleepy. A large number of MVAs may be considered work or occupational accidents. Some groups of professionals are particularly at risk, such as truck drivers and bus drivers, who often cumulate several risk factors for driving while sleepy: night-shift work, long periods of work, insufficient environmental conditions to get restorative sleep, and sleep disorders such as OSA. It is, therefore, difficult to separate formally the cost of accidents at the workplace from the cost of accidents in the entire population. The only estimate in the field to the authors' knowledge was made in Australia, where the adjusted prevalence of work injuries due to EDS was estimated to be 60,681 cases in 2016 to 2017. Thus, the health system costs attributed to inadequate sleep were estimated to be $620 million.[27]

Besides this single estimate, multiple reports have clearly shown how professional drivers were concerned about being sleepy at the wheel.

In Brazil, a recent survey was performed in 670 professional male truck drivers, with a mean age of 41.9 (±11.1) years. The prevalence of sleepiness while driving was 31.5%. The following working conditions were significantly associated with sleepiness while driving regardless of other working or behavioral characteristics, age, and sleep duration:

- A distance from the last shipment of more than 1000 km (odds ratio [OR] = 1.54)
- A formal labor contract with a productivity-based salary (OR = 2.65)[37]

In Sweden, it has also been shown that shift-working bus drivers frequently struggle to stay awake and thus countermeasures are needed in order to guarantee safe driving with split-shift schedules.[38] It is not certain, however, that professional drivers are sufficiently aware of the risk of driving while sleepy. Three hundred Australian drivers recently completed a questionnaire that assessed crash risk perceptions for sleepy driving, drink driving, and speeding. Additionally, the participants' perceptions of crash risk were assessed for 5 different contextual scenarios that included different levels of sleepiness (low and high), driving

duration (short and long), and time of day/circadian influences (afternoon and nighttime) on driving. The analysis confirmed that sleepy driving was considered a risky driving behavior but not as risky as high levels of speed ($P<.05$). The results suggest a lack of awareness or appreciation of circadian rhythm functioning, in particular the descending phase of circadian rhythm that promotes increased sleepiness in the afternoon and during the early hours of the morning.[39]

Besides accidents at work, a larger group, again of professionals, are simply using their car to go to work, and accidents on the way to and/or back from work are considered in many countries as occupational or work accidents. Due to urban development and the need for larger homes outside city centers, workers are driving more and more every day and, therefore, reducing their sleep time, which is one of the determinants of sleep debt around the world. The farther they live from work, the less they sleep, the longer they drive, and the higher the risk of sleepiness-related accidents. In a specific survey enquiring about sleeping at the wheel on French highways, with the same questionnaire used in regular highway drivers (2196 in 1996 and 3545 in 2011), it has been shown that drivers have reduced their mean weekly sleep duration over 15 years and have a higher risk of sleepiness at the wheel.[40]

Public Accidents

The media frequently report on spectacular public accidents in which sleepiness is considered a significant risk factor.

Decades ago, the National Commission on Sleep Disorders Research in the United States highlighted the role of sleepiness in several environmental health disasters in history,[41] including

- The Three Mile Island nuclear power plant incident, which occurred at 4:00 AM; overnight shift workers failed to respond quickly because they were sleepy.
- The nuclear plant disaster at Chernobyl, which took place at 1:30 AM, also is linked to human error influenced by sleepiness.
- Sleep loss is thought to have played a role in the Exxon Valdez oil tanker spill and the Space Shuttle Challenger accident (where managers at the flight center were known to be working irregular hours on very little sleep). These and other accidents, both small scale and large scale, highlight the potentially devastating consequences of being drowsy or sleeping at the wheel or on security monotonous conditions.

Fatigue and sleepiness in airplane pilots also are crucial issues because they face jet lag, long extended shifts, and sometimes stressful climate conditions.[42,43] No specific cost has been reported, however, to the authors' knowledge, on piloting while sleepy and associated accident risk.

REFERENCES

1. Leger D. The cost of sleep related accidents. A report for the National Commission on Sleep Disorders Research. Sleep 1994;17:84–93.
2. Goncalves M, Amici R, Lucas R, et al. Sleepiness at the wheel across Europe: a survey of 19 countries. J Sleep Res 2015;24:242–53.
3. Komada Y, Nishida Y, Namba K, et al. Elevated risk of motor vehicle accident for male drivers with obstructive sleep apnea syndrome in the Tokyo metropolitan area. Tohoku J Exp Med 2009; 219:11–6.
4. Honn KA, Van Dongen HPA, Dawson D. Working Time Society consensus statements: prescriptive rule sets and risk management-based approaches for the management of fatigue-related risk in working time arrangements. Ind Health 2019;57:264–80.
5. McCartt AT, Rohrbaugh JW, Hammer MC, et al. Factors associated with falling asleep at the wheel among long-distance truck drivers. Accid Anal Prev 2000;32:493–504.
6. Leger D, du Roscoat E, Bayon V, et al. Short sleep in young adults: is it insomnia or sleep debt? Prevalence and clinical description of short sleep in a representative sample of 1004 young adults from France. Sleep Med 2011;12:454–62.
7. Klerman EB, Dijk DJ. Interindividual variation in sleep duration and its association with sleep debt in young adults. Sleep 2005;28:1253–9.
8. Wang F, Chow IHI, Li L, et al. Sleep duration and patterns in Chinese patients with diabetes: a meta-analysis of comparative studies and epidemiological surveys. Perspect Psychiatr Care 2019;55:344–53.
9. Vedaa Ø, Harris A, Erevik EK, et al. Short rest between shifts (quick returns) and night work is associated with work-related accidents. Int Arch Occup Environ Health 2019;92:829–35.
10. Berneking M, Rosen IM, Kirsch DB, et al, American Academy of Sleep Medicine Board of Directors. The risk of fatigue and sleepiness in the ridesharing industry: an American Academy of Sleep Medicine Position statement. J Clin Sleep Med 2018;14:683–5.
11. Liang Y, Horrey WJ, Howard ME, et al. Prediction of drowsiness events in night shift workers during morning driving. Accid Anal Prev 2019;126:105–14.
12. McHill AW, Hull JT, Wang W, et al. Chronic sleep curtailment, even without extended (>16-h) wakefulness, degrades human vigilance performance. Proc Natl Acad Sci U S A 2018;115:6070–5.
13. Anund A, Ahlström C, Fors C, et al. Are professional drivers less sleepy than non-professional drivers? Scand J Work Environ Health 2018;44:88–95.
14. Mollicone D, Kan K, Mott C, et al. Predicting performance and safety based on driver fatigue. Accid Anal Prev 2019;126:142–5.
15. Foss RD, Smith RL, O'Brien NP. School start times and teenage driver motor vehicle crashes. Accid Anal Prev 2019;126:54–63.
16. Nuutinen T, Roos E, Ray C, et al. Computer use, sleep duration and health symptoms: a cross-sectional study of 15-year-olds in three countries. Int J Public Health 2014;59:619–28.
17. Meyer C, Ferrari Junior GJ, Andrade RD, et al. Factors associated with excessive daytime sleepiness among Brazilian adolescents. Chronobiol Int 2019; 12:1–9.
18. Léger D, Bayon V, Ohayon MM, et al. Insomnia and accidents: cross sectional study (EQUINOX) on sleep-related home, work and car accidents in 5293 subjects with insomnia from ten countries. J Sleep Res 2014;23:143–52.
19. Rizzo D, Libman E, Creti L, et al. Determinants of policy decisions for non-commercial drivers with OSA: an integrative review. Sleep Med Rev 2018; 37:130–7.
20. Bayon V, Philip P, LegerD. Socio-professional handicap and accidental risk in patients with Hypersomnias of Central Origin. Sleep Med Rev 2009;13:421–6.
21. Road Travel. Road safety facts in: Association for Safe International. 2019. Available at: https://www.asirt.org/safe-travel/road-safety-facts/. Accessed July 15, 2019.
22. Cost Data and Prevention Policies | Motor Vehicle Safety | CDC Injury National Health Transportation Safety Administration (NHTSA). 2016. Available at: https://www.cdc.gov/motorvehiclesafety/costs/index.htmlaccidents cost. Accessed July 15, 2019.
23. Wijnen W, Weijermars W, Vanden Berghe W, et al. Crash cost estimates for European countries, deliverable 3.2 of the H2020 project SafetyCube. Loughborough (England): Loughborough University, SafetyCube; 2017. Available at: https://dspace.lboro.ac.uk/dspace-jspui/bitstream/2134/24949/1/D32-CrashCostEstimates_Final.pdf. Accessed July 15, 2019.
24. Horne J, Reyner LA. Sleep related vehicle accidents. BMJ 1995;310:565–7.
25. Dawson A, Reid K. Fatigue, alcohol, and performance impairment. Nature 1997;388:235–7.
26. Blincoe LJ, Miller TR, Zaloshnja E, et al. National Highway Traffic Safety Administration. The economic and societal impact of motor vehicle crashes, (revised) (Report no. DOT HS 812 013) 2015. Washington, DC. Available at: https://crashstats.nhtsa.dot.gov/Api/Public/ViewPublication/812013. Accessed July 15, 2019.

27. Bruck D. Asleep on the job: costs of inadequate sleep in Australia, Deloitte access economics 2017. p. 95p. Available at: https://www.sleephealthfoundation.org.au/files/Asleep_on_the_job/Asleep_on_the_Job_SHF_report-WEB_small.pdf. Accessed July 15, 2019.

28. de Mello MT, Bittencourt LR, Cunha Rde C, et al. Sleep and transit in Brazil: new legislation. J Clin Sleep Med 2009;5:164–6.

29. Frost & Sullivan. Hidden health crisis costing America billions. Underdiagnosing and undertreating obstructive sleep apnea draining healthcare system. Darien (IL): American Academy of Sleep Medicine; 2016. Available at: http://www.aasmnet.org/sleep-apnea-economic-impact.aspx. Accessed July 15, 2019.

30. Frost & Sullivan. In an age of constant activity, the solution to improving the nation's health may lie in helping it sleep better. What benefits do patients experience in treating their obstructive sleep apnea? Darien (IL): American Academy of Sleep Medicine; 2016. Available at: http://www.aasmnet.org/sleep-apnea-economic-impact.aspx. Accessed July 15, 2019.

31. AASM. Sleepy driving highly prevalent among college students 2019. Available at: https://aasm.org/sleepy-driving-highly-prevalent-among-college-students/. Accessed July 15, 2019.

32. Merill D. No one values your life more than the Federal government 29-10-2017. Available at: https://www.bloomberg.com/graphics/2017-value-of-life/. Accessed July 15, 2019.

33. Kip-Viscusi W. Pricing lives. Guideposts for a safer society. Princeton (NJ): Pricetown University Education Editions; 2018. p. 296. Ebook.

34. Anderson NJ, Smith CK, Byrd JL. Work-related injury factors and safety climate perception in truck drivers. Am J Ind Med 2017;60:711–23.

35. Ferguson SA, Appleton SL, Reynolds AC, et al. Making errors at work due to sleepiness or sleep problems is not confined to non-standard work hours: results of the 2016 Sleep Health Foundation national survey. Chronobiol Int 2019;36:758–69.

36. Redeker NS, Caruso CC, Hashmi SD, et al. Workplace Interventions to promote sleep health and an alert, healthy workforce. J Clin Sleep Med 2019;15:649–57.

37. Girotto E, Bortoletto MSS, González AD, et al. Working conditions and sleepiness while driving among truck drivers. Traffic Inj Prev 2019;20:504–9.

38. Anund A, Fors C, Ihlström J, et al. An on-road study of sleepiness in split shifts among city bus drivers. Accid Anal Prev 2018;114:71–6.

39. Watling CN, Armstrong KA, Smith SS, et al. Crash risk perception of sleepy driving and its comparisons with drink driving and speeding: which behavior is perceived as the riskiest? Traffic Inj Prev 2016;17:400–5.

40. Quera-Salva MA, Hartley S, Sauvagnac-Quera R, et al. Association between reported sleep need and sleepiness at the wheel: comparative study on French highways between 1996 and 2011. BMJ Open 2016;6(12):e012382.

41. National Commission on Sleep Disorders Research (U.S.). Wake up America [microform]: a National sleep alert: report of the National Commission on Sleep Disorders Research/submitted to the United States Congress and to the secretary. Washington, DC: U.S. Department of Health and Human Services; 1995.

42. Sallinen M, Åkerstedt T, Härmä M, et al. Recurrent on-duty sleepiness and alertness management strategies in long-Haul airline pilots. Aerosp Med Hum Perform 2018;89:601–8.

43. Cosgrave J, Wu LJ, van den Berg M, et al. Sleep on long Haul layovers and pilot fatigue at the start of the next duty period. Aerosp Med Hum Perform 2018;89:19–25.

Sleep Apnea, Sleepiness, and Driving Risk

Maria R. Bonsignore, MD, FERS[a,b,*], Oreste Marrone, MD[b], Francesco Fanfulla, MD[c]

KEYWORDS

- Obstructive sleep apnea • Epidemiology • Pathophysiology • Subjective sleepiness
- Objective sleepiness • CPAP

KEY POINTS

- Obstructive sleep apnea is often associated with excessive daytime sleepiness and increases the risk of driving accidents.
- Treatment with continuous positive airway pressure normalizes the risk of driving accidents in patients with obstructive sleep apnea.
- Many studies have analyzed clinical factors associated with sleepiness in obstructive sleep apnea to identify patients at high risk of driving accidents.
- Subjective sleepiness (Epworth Sleepiness Scale score) is a slightly better predictor of driving accidents in obstructive sleep apnea than objective sleepiness assessed by multiple sleep latency test.
- Other tests, such as the maintenance of wakefulness test or driving simulation, may help to predict driving risk.

OBSTRUCTIVE SLEEP APNEA

Obstructive sleep apnea (OSA) is highly prevalent in the general population, especially in obese patients.[1] OSA occurs at all ages, is more frequent in males, and is often associated with hypertension and other comorbidities.[2]

OSA is characterized by partial or complete collapse of the upper airway during sleep. During airway obstruction, increasing respiratory efforts occur until an increase in airway dilator muscle tone reestablishes upper airway patency. The cycle can occur hundreds of times during the night. The most common clinical symptoms of OSA are intermittent loud snoring, excessive daytime sleepiness (EDS), and unrefreshing sleep.[2]

The diagnosis of OSA requires polysomnography or cardiorespiratory monitoring during sleep.[3,4] Pretest probability of OSA can be assessed by questionnaires,[5,6] but a sleep recording is necessary to diagnose OSA and assess its severity. The apnea–hypopnea index (AHI), that is, the frequency of respiratory events, is used to define OSA severity. OSA is classified as mild, moderate, or severe according to AHI of 5 to less than 15 per hour, between 15 and 30 per hour, and more than 30 per hour, respectively.[2] AHI does not discriminate OSA physiologic or clinical phenotypes,[7] and other metrics are considered in daily clinical practice, such as hypoxemia during sleep.[8]

Intermittent hypoxia and sleep fragmentation are the main pathophysiological features of OSA.

Disclosure Statement: No commercial or financial interest to disclose by any of the authors.

[a] Respiratory Division, Dipartimento di Promozione Della Salute, Materno-Infantile, Medicina Interna e Specialistica di Eccellenza "G. D'Alessandro" (PROMISE), University of Palermo, Palermo, Italy; [b] Istituto per la Ricerca e l'Innovazione Biomedica (IRIB), National Research Council (CNR), Via Ugo La Malfa 153, Palermo 90146, Italy; [c] Respiratory Function and Sleep Medicine Unit, Istituti Clinici Scientifici Maugeri IRCCS, Via Maugeri 4, Pavia 27100, Italy

* Corresponding author. Respiratory Division, PROMISE Department, University of Palermo, Piazza delle Cliniche, 2, Palermo 90100, Italy.

E-mail address: marisa.bonsignore@irib.cnr.it

Sleep Med Clin 14 (2019) 431–439
https://doi.org/10.1016/j.jsmc.2019.08.001
1556-407X/19/© 2019 Elsevier Inc. All rights reserved.

OSA exerts detrimental effects on health, including cardiometabolic diseases, and accidents while driving or at work.[2] Cognitive dysfunction, investigated in recent years by highly sophisticated methodologies,[9,10] could contribute to driving risk, but studies are still lacking.

Continuous positive airway pressure (CPAP) is the standard treatment of OSA, especially in moderate and severe cases.[11,12] By splinting the upper airway open, CPAP prevents obstructive events during sleep, and their acute and long-term negative consequences.[13] CPAP needs to be manually or automatically titrated in each patient to establish its therapeutic level.[12] Patients should use CPAP every time they sleep, but adherence to treatment is often suboptimal, especially in patients without EDS.[14] CPAP devices allow the download of data regarding daily use, and good compliance is considered 4 hours or more for at least 70% of the nights. Other treatments for OSA, such as positional therapies, mandibular advancement devices or upper airway surgery, are not discussed here because their effect on driving risk remains unknown.

SLEEPINESS IN OBSTRUCTIVE SLEEP APNEA

The prevalence of subjective EDS in patients with OSA is less than 50%. In the Analysis of the European Sleep Apnea Database (ESADA) study, only 44.4% of participants with suspected OSA reported EDS.[15] Similarly, in the Icelandic Sleep Cohort, the prevalence of EDS was 42.6%.[16] EDS prevalence is low in patients with heart failure and OSA,[17] although it is relatively high in asthmatic patients with OSA,[18] indicating that EDS varies with the occurrence of comorbidities.

Predictors of EDS in patients with OSA may help to identify patients at high risk of driving accidents. Many studies[19–49] show variability in characteristics and sample size, methodology used for OSA diagnosis, and sleepiness assessment tools (**Table 1**). Subjective sleepiness was assessed in the majority of studies by using the Epworth Sleepiness Scale (ESS) questionnaire.[50] Other simpler questionnaires, based on positive response to 2 out of 3 questions (feeling sleepy sitting quietly; feeling tired, fatigued, or sleepy; having trouble staying awake) have also been used.[21] Other studies indicate that a positive response to the simple question: "Are you sleepy while driving?" is highly predictive of car accidents. However, the reliability of questionnaires is limited.

Objective tests, such as the multiple sleep latency test (MSLT) and the maintenance of wakefulness test have been used less extensively, and their clinical utility has been challenged.[51] The maintenance of wakefulness test is considered more appropriate than MSLT in reflecting the ability to remain awake during monotonous driving in patients with OSA, especially when its duration is prolonged to 40 minutes.[52]

Results of studies assessing predictors of subjective and objective sleepiness in OSA are reported in **Tables 2** and **3**, respectively. Positive relationships resulting mostly from multiple regression are reported. A role for the AHI or oxygen desaturation during sleep in predicting sleepiness was reported by some but not all studies. Sleepiness was associated with prolonged sleep times in some studies, possibly reflecting the increased

Table 1 Characteristics of studies on sleepiness in OSA		
Population	General population	3 studies[19–21]
	Sleep clinics	28 studies[22–49]
Sample size	<400 (range 40–355)	19 studies[23–28,31,33,35–38,40–43,46,47,49]
	>500 (range 518–16,583, not all used PSG)	12 studies[19–22,29,30,32,34,39,44,45,48]
Diagnostic method	Full PSG	28 studies[19–22,24–46]
	Oximetry from PSG	2 studies[47,48]
	Polygraphy	1 study[49]
Participants	OSA (no AHI range restriction)	25 studies[19,21–27,29–31,33–37,39–42,44–46,48,49]
	OSA (AHI ≥15 or ≥30 required)	6 studies[20,28,32,38,43,47]
Sleepiness assessment tool	ESS	19 studies[24,27,29–34,37–39,41,43–49]
	MSLT	2 studies[22,26]
	EDS by combined ESS and MSLT	6 studies[25,28,35,36,40,42]
	Other subjective tests	4 studies[19–21,41]
	Other objective tests	2 studies[23,24]

Abbreviations: ESS, Epworth Sleepiness Scale; MSLT, multiple sleep latency test; PSG, polysomnography.

Table 2
Summary of results of studies on predictors of subjective sleepiness in OSA

Sleep duration/ structure	Long TST/high sleep efficiency	4 studies[28,29,36,43]
	Arousals/sleep fragmentation	5 studies[24,29,31,32,36]
Nocturnal hypoxemia	SaO$_2$ levels and/or SaO$_2$ dips	9 studies[28,32,34,36,38,45,47–49]
AHI		10 studies[20,25,27,29,30,32,34,36,44,49]
Metabolism	Insulin resistance, diabetes, adipokines	4 studies[19,30,42,43]
Obesity or body mass index		7 studies[19,22,30,32,34,44,46]
Depression		7 studies[19,21,30,33,38,39,44]
Age		4 studies[19,27,29,45]
Miscellanea	Habitual sleep duration	2 studies[19,20]
	Smoking	1 study[19]
	Insomnia symptoms	1 study[20]
	Nocturia	1 study[21]
	Respiratory effort	1 study[23]
	PLM	1 study[46]
	Hypertension	1 study[46]

Abbreviation: TST, total sleep time.

sleep pressure associated with poor sleep quality. However, sleep fragmentation predicted sleepiness in a minority of studies. Conversely, obesity or metabolic variables were often associated with sleepiness,[53,54] and depression may exert an independent role in EDS pathogenesis. Overall, sleepiness in patients with OSA seems to be multifactorial, and no single clinical or polysomnographic variable, or combination of different factors, can be used to predict sleepiness at the wheel and risk of car accidents.

OBSTRUCTIVE SLEEP APNEA AND DRIVING RISK

Fatigue or sleep-related accidents represent a common cause of traffic accidents,[55–57] with a variable proportion of accidents attributable to sleepiness.[55,58,59] Ten percent to 30% of fatal accidents have been attributed to sleepiness at wheel,[60,61] and car crashes related to falling asleep often cause death and severe injury.[62] Death of the driver occurred in 11.4% of sleepiness-related accidents, in contrast with 5.6% of accidents unrelated to sleep.[63] Sleepiness-related motor vehicle accidents (MVA) may result from falling asleep while driving and behavior impairment attributable to sleepiness.[64]

The third edition of the *International Classification of Sleep Disorders* defines daytime sleepiness as the inability to stay awake and alert during the major waking episodes of the day, resulting in periods of irrepressible need for sleep or unintended lapses into drowsiness or sleep.[65] Sleepiness may vary in severity and is more likely to occur in sedentary, boring, and monotonous situations that require little active participation. Some patients are aware of increasing sleepiness before

Table 3
Summary of results of studies on predictors of objective sleepiness OSA

Sleep duration/structure	Long TST/high sleep efficiency	3 studies[26,28,36]
	Arousals/sleep fragmentation	4 studies[24,26,35,36]
Nocturnal hypoxemia	SaO$_2$ levels and/or SaO$_2$ dips	5 studies[22,23,28,35,36]
AHI		1 study[25]
Humoral factors	Cytokines, hormones, metabolism	2 studies[40,42]
Miscellanea	Daytime Paco$_2$	1 study[23]
	ESS	1 study[25]
	Snoring	1 study[26]

Abbreviation: TST, total sleep time.

falling asleep, whereas others can fall asleep with little or no prodromal symptoms.[66] Drivers may be unaware of having lapses, but are aware of loss of vehicle control during out-of-lane excursion.[67]

Behavioral sleepiness is defined as difficulty in remaining awake even while participants are performing activities.[68] Sleepiness at the wheel is defined as difficulty in remaining awake or episodes of drowsiness interfering with driving skills[60]; alternatively, a driver can be defined as being habitually sleepy if he or she became so sleepy while driving that he or she feared falling asleep, and if this severe sleepiness while driving occurred at least once every 3 times he or she drove on a highway.[69]

Sleepiness at the wheel is frequent in the general population. Episodes of sleepiness at the wheel in the previous 2 years were reported by 17% of European drivers.[70] It can be caused by sleep disorders, including sleep apnea, but also by sleep deprivation, shift work, or nonrestorative sleep.[60] Two studies reported a prevalence of 3.6% of habitually sleepy drivers in the general population.[69,71] In other studies, the prevalence of sleepiness at the wheel ranged from 1.1% to 58%.[60]

Insufficient sleep is a major factor in MVA.[72–75] Participants with very short (≤5 hours) or short (6 hours) sleep duration were at risk for drowsy driving in one report.[71] A population-based questionnaire survey found that male gender, office or manual labor, the presence of EDS, depression, habitual snoring, and perceived insufficient sleep were independent risk factors for drowsy driving.[76] The score of the ESS was higher in habitually sleepy drivers, but only 50% reported overall EDS, defined an ESS of greater than 9.[69] Participants are able to perceive sleepiness under conditions of acute sleep deprivation, but this ability, and the ability to perceive performance deficits, reach a plateau in the presence of chronic sleep insufficiency.[77]

In contrast, other physiologic or individual factors should be taken into account, such as circadian or homeostatic effects, time on task duration, or fatigue. Recently, the effect of light conditions had an independent effect on driver sleepiness with worse performance during darkness.[78]

The association between self-reported sleepiness at the wheel and risk of MVA has been investigated in a recent meta-analysis,[60] with a pooled odds ratio of 2.51 (95% confidence interval, 1.87–3.39). However, larger studies report a lower increase in risk that was not related to methodologic issues. Recently, a dose–response relationship was shown between driver's sleep

in the past 24 hours and the risk of causing an MVA.[79] Drivers who reported having slept for 6, 5, or 4 hours or less in the 24 hours before crashing had odds ratio of 1.3, 1.9, 2.9, and 15.1, respectively, of having been culpable for their crashes compared with drivers who reported 7 to 9 hours of sleep.[79]

OSA contributes to the occurrence of EDS and MVA (**Table 4**). In a meta-analysis by Ellen and colleagues,[80] drivers with OSA were at risk of involvement in MVAs. However, an association between crash risk and daytime sleepiness or OSA severity was found in a minority of studies, leading the authors to state "clinicians should be cautious in using the presence or absence of this symptom as the sole factor in determining the fitness to drive of patients with sleep apnea."[80] Subsequent meta-analyses[81,82] reported similar results. Commercial drivers may be at particularly high risk of MVA because of increased exposure, but the risk could not be precisely assessed based on OSA severity, or subjective and objective sleepiness.[81] More recently, Garbarino and colleagues[82] analyzed the risk of occupational accidents including MVAs in commercial drivers, and the effect size was found to be larger in them compared with other workers with OSA.

A cohort study assessed the risk on MVA in North American police officers according to risk for different sleep disorders.[83] Screening was positive in 33.6% of police officers for OSA, in 6.5% for insomnia, and in 5.4% for shift work disorder. Participants who screened positive for at least 1 sleep disorder, however, reported similar rates of episodes of falling asleep while driving as control participants (17.9% vs 12.7%). Such low sensitivity may be explained by the screening strategy used, as opposed to actual diagnosis of sleep disorders.

In a large Swedish study, only severe EDS (ESS ≥16), but not OSA severity, was associated with increased risk of MVA[84]; driving distance (exposure to risk), short habitual sleep time (≤5 hours/night) and use of hypnotics also predicted risk. Analysis of the European Sleep Apnea Database showed that at least 1 risk factor was present in 68.7% and 51.3% of male and female drivers, respectively.[85] Predictors of MVA were severe EDS (ESS ≥16), age, female sex, body mass index, AHI, and driving distance of more than 15,000 km/y. Of interest, the mean sum of MVA risk factors increased with OSA severity and was higher in males than in females.

Although the role of OSA in increasing the risk for MVA can be considered evidence based, several problems remain. For example, the large

Table 4
Summary of results of meta-analyses on risk of MVA in patients with OSA, and effects of CPAP treatment

Author, Year, Ref	Study Type	Studies	Results
Ellen et al,[80] 2006	Systematic review of literature until 2006	30 studies, 27 in noncommercial drivers, 3 in commercial drivers	Increased risk of MVA in OSA. Studies did not consistently find that sleepiness and OSA severity were correlated with crash risk.
Tregear et al,[81] 2009	Systematic review and meta-analysis (until May 2009)	18 retrospective studies, 2 in commercial drivers	Crash rate associated with OSA between 1.21 and 4.89. Predictors of risk: body mass index, AHI, oxygen saturation. ESS not significant. No control for exposure in most studies, and significant heterogeneity.
Garbarino et al,[91] 2016	Systematic review and meta-analysis (until Sept 2015)	10 studies (7 in the meta-analysis) on occupational accidents including professional driving	Increased risk in patients with OSA (OR, 2.18; 95% CI, 1.53–3.10). Risk associated with driving higher compared with other occupational activities.
Tregear et al,[88] 2010	Systematic review and meta-analysis (until May 2009)	9 observational studies on effects of CPAP	CPAP decrease the risk for accidents in patients with OSA (RR, 0.28; 95% CI, 0.22–0.35). ESS decreased after 1 night of CPAP and driving performance improved after 2–7 d of treatment.
Antonopoulos et al,[89] 2011	Meta-analysis (until July 2011)	10 studies on MVA, 5 studies on near miss accidents, 6 studies on performance at driving simulator	CPAP reduced the risk of real (OR, 0.21; 95% CI, 0.12–0.35) and near-miss (OR, 0.09; 95% CI, 0.04–0.21) accidents in patients with OSA, and improved performance at simulated driving (OR, 0.09; 95% CI, 0.04–0.21).
Patil et al,[13] 2019	Meta-analysis on effects of CPAP in several domains, including driving risk (until April 2015)	4 RCTs on driving simulator performance, 10 studies on MVA in noncommercial drivers	No improvement in performance at driving simulators in RCTs. Significant reduction in car accident risk after CPAP (OR, 0.09; 95% CI, 0.04–0.21)

Abbreviations: CI, confidence interval; OR, odds ratio; RCT, randomized, controlled trial; RR, risk ratio.

majority of individuals studied were men, whereas MVA risk in women is insufficiently studied to date. Similarly, elderly patients with OSA may show a higher risk, compensated by a low driving distance per year and/or preventive behaviors such as avoiding driving at night. In contrast, commercial drivers often drive heavy trucks, besides driving long distances. Furthermore, it was recently estimated that OSA could be held responsible for only about 7% of total MVAs.[86]

THE EFFECTS OF CONTINUOUS POSITIVE AIRWAY PRESSURE TREATMENT ON DRIVING RISK IN OBSTRUCTIVE SLEEP APNEA

Studies agree on the positive effect of OSA treatment in reducing the risk of MVA (see **Table 4**). The first meta-analysis on the effects of CPAP also calculated that costs of OSA-associated MVAs were far higher than cost of OSA treatment.[87] Tregear and colleagues[88] confirmed a significant risk reduction following OSA treatment (risk ratio, 0.28; 95% confidence interval, 0.22–0.35; P<.001). EDS improved significantly after a single night, and simulated driving performance improved significantly within 2 to 7 days of CPAP treatment.[88] Not only MVA, but also near-miss accidents, decreased with CPAP, and performance at simulated driving improved in treated patients.[89] Finally, the meta-analysis recently published by Patil and colleagues[13] confirmed that CPAP treatment effectively decreased both EDS and MVAs.

Compliance with CPAP treatment remains a major problem. In a cohort of truck drivers, participants with OSA nonadherent to CPAP had a 5-fold greater crash rate compared with controls without OSA; the crash rate was similar in fully adherent drivers and controls.[90] Nonadherent drivers remained highly dangerous, because information on their health status could not be communicated to other employers owing to privacy regulations. Moreover, sleep deprivation is frequent in commercial drivers and increased the risk of accidents, although it can be prevented by naps,[91] emphasizing the importance of preventive measures. The American Academy of Sleep Medicine has recently issued a document specifically regarding the management of OSA in commercial motor vehicle operators.[92]

SUMMARY

The evaluation of fitness to drive in patients with OSA is a current problem worldwide. The European Union has updated the rules on driving license regulations,[93] and OSA was included among disorders for which the evaluation of fitness to drive is mandatory. Application of the European Union Directive, however, would require reliable tools to evaluate the risk of MVA,[94] which are currently missing. A lack of consensus in clinicians' judgment of fitness to drive is common for both untreated and CPAP-treated patients with OSA.[95]

Adherence to CPAP is poor in many patients with OSA, but the effect on driving risk of alternative treatments for OSA, such as mandibular advancement devices or positional treatment,

has been little investigated. One short-term randomized controlled study reported similar positive effects of CPAP and mandibular advancement devices on sleepiness and driving performance,[96] but data on actual MVAs after long-term treatment are needed.[97] Driving regulations should be updated to ensure safety on the road and counteract irresponsible behaviors, especially by commercial drivers.

REFERENCES

1. Senaratna CV, Perret JL, Lodge CJ, et al. Prevalence of obstructive sleep apnea in the general population: a systematic review. Sleep Med Rev 2017;34: 70–81.
2. Lévy P, Kohler M, McNicholas WT, et al. Obstructive sleep apnoea syndrome. Nat Rev Dis Primers 2015; 1:15015.
3. Kapur VK, Auckley DH, Chowdhuri S, et al. Clinical practice guideline for diagnostic testing for adult obstructive sleep apnea: an American Academy of Sleep Medicine Clinical Practice Guideline. J Clin Sleep Med 2017;13(3):479–504.
4. Gamaldo C, Buenaver L, Chernyshev O, et al, OSA assessment tools task force of the American Academy of Sleep Medicine. Evaluation of clinical tools to screen and assess for obstructive sleep apnea. J Clin Sleep Med 2018;14:1239–44.
5. Chiu HY, Chen PY, Chuang LP, et al. Diagnostic accuracy of the Berlin questionnaire, STOP-BANG, STOP, and Epworth sleepiness scale in detecting obstructive sleep apnea: a bivariate meta-analysis. Sleep Med Rev 2017;36:57–70.
6. Rosen IM, Kirsch DB, Carden KA, et al, American Academy of Sleep Medicine Board of Directors. Clinical use of a home sleep apnea test: an updated American Academy of Sleep Medicine Position Statement. J Clin Sleep Med 2018;14:2075–7.
7. Zinchuk AV, Gentry MJ, Concato J, et al. Phenotypes in obstructive sleep apnea: a definition, examples and evolution of approaches. Sleep Med Rev 2017;35:113–23.
8. Chen F, Chen K, Zhang C, et al. Evaluating the clinical value of the hypoxia burden index in patients with obstructive sleep apnea. Postgrad Med 2018; 130:436–41.
9. Leng Y, McEvoy CT, Allen IE, et al. Association of sleep-disordered breathing with cognitive function and risk of cognitive impairment: a systematic review and meta-analysis. JAMA Neurol 2017;74: 1237–45.
10. Polsek D, Gildeh N, Cash D, et al. Obstructive sleep apnoea and Alzheimer's disease: in search of shared pathomechanisms. Neurosci Biobehav Rev 2018;86:142–9.

11. Sullivan CE. Nasal positive airway pressure and sleep apnea. Reflections on an experimental method that became a therapy. Am J Respir Crit Care Med 2018;198:581–7.

12. Patil SP, Ayappa IA, Caples SM, et al. Treatment of adult obstructive sleep apnea with positive airway pressure: an American Academy of Sleep Medicine Clinical Practice Guideline. J Clin Sleep Med 2019; 15(2):335–43.

13. Patil SP, Ayappa IA, Caples SM, et al. Treatment of adult obstructive sleep apnea with positive airway pressure: an American Academy of Sleep Medicine systematic review, meta-analysis, and GRADE assessment. J Clin Sleep Med 2019;15: 301–34.

14. Mehrtash M, Bakker JP, Ayas N. Predictors of continuous positive airway pressure adherence in patients with obstructive sleep apnea. Lung 2019. https://doi.org/10.1007/s00408-018-00193-1.

15. Saaresranta T, Hedner J, Bonsignore MR, et al, ESADA Study Group. Clinical phenotypes and co-morbidity in European sleep apnoea patients. PLoS One 2016;11:e0163439.

16. Ye L, Pien GW, Ratcliffe SJ, et al. The different clinical faces of obstructive sleep apnoea: a cluster analysis. Eur Respir J 2014;44:1600–7.

17. Pak VM, Strouss L, Yaggi HK, et al. Mechanisms of reduced sleepiness symptoms in heart failure and obstructive sleep apnea. J Sleep Res 2018;28: e12778.

18. Bonsignore MR, Pepin JL, Anttalainen U, et al, ESADA Study Group. Clinical presentation of patients with suspected obstructive sleep apnea and self-reported physician-diagnosed asthma in the ESADA cohort. J Sleep Res 2018;27(6):e12729.

19. Bixler EO, Vgontzas AN, Lin HM, et al. Excessive daytime sleepiness in a general population sample: the role of sleep apnea, age, obesity, diabetes, and depression. J Clin Endocrinol Metab 2005;90: 4510–5.

20. Kapur VK, Baldwin CM, Resnick HE, et al. Sleepiness in patients with moderate to severe sleep-disordered breathing. Sleep 2005;28:472–7.

21. Adams RJ, Appleton SL, Vakulin A, et al. Association of daytime sleepiness with obstructive sleep apnoea and comorbidities varies by sleepiness definition in a population cohort of men. Respirology 2016;21:1314–21.

22. Mendelson WB. The relationship of sleepiness and blood pressure to respiratory variables in obstructive sleep apnea. Chest 1995;108:966–72.

23. Zamagni M, Sforza E, Boudewijns A, et al. Respiratory effort. A factor contributing to sleep propensity in patients with obstructive sleep apnea. Chest 1996;109:651–8.

24. Bennett LS, Langford BA, Stradling JR, et al. Sleep fragmentation indices as predictors of daytime sleepiness and nCPAP response in obstructive

25. Leng PH, Low SY, Hsu A, et al. The clinical predictors of sleepiness correlated with the Multiple Sleep Latency Test in an Asian Singapore population: predictors of sleepiness. Sleep 2003;26:878–81.

26. Seneviratne U, Puvenendran K. Excessive daytime sleepiness in obstructive sleep apnea: prevalence, severity, and predictors. Sleep Med 2004;5:339–43.

27. Goncalves MA, Paiva T, Ramos E, et al. Obstructive sleep apnea syndrome, sleepiness, and quality of life. Chest 2004;125:2091–6.

28. Mediano O, Barceló A, de la Peña M, et al. Daytime sleepiness and polysomnographic variables in sleep apnoea patients. Eur Respir J 2007;30:110–3.

29. Roure N, Gomez S, Mediano O, et al. Daytime sleepiness and polysomnography in obstructive sleep apnea patients. Sleep Med 2008;9:727–31.

30. Koutsourelakis I, Perraki E, Bonakis A, et al. Determinants of subjective sleepiness in suspected obstructive sleep apnoea. J Sleep Res 2008;17:437–43.

31. Bausmer U, Gouveris H, Selivanova O, et al. Correlation of the Epworth Sleepiness Scale with respiratory sleep parameters in patients with sleep-related breathing disorders and upper airway pathology. Eur Arch Otorhinolaryngol 2010;267:1645–8.

32. Oksenberg A, Arons E, Nasser K, et al. Severe obstructive sleep apnea: sleepy versus nonsleepy patients. Laryngoscope 2010;120:643–8.

33. Ishman SL, Cavey RM, Mettel TL, et al. Depression, sleepiness, and disease severity in patients with obstructive sleep apnea. Laryngoscope 2010;120: 2331–5.

34. Chen R, Xiong K, Lian Y, et al. Daytime sleepiness and its determining factors in Chinese obstructive sleep apnea patients. Sleep Breath 2011;15:129–35.

35. Sun Y, Ning Y, Huang L, et al. Polysomnographic characteristics of daytime sleepiness in obstructive sleep apnea syndrome. Sleep Breath 2012;16: 375–81.

36. Cai S, Chen R, Zhang Y, et al. Correlation of Epworth Sleepiness Scale with multiple sleep latency test and its diagnostic accuracy in assessing excessive daytime sleepiness in patients with obstructive sleep apnea hypopnea syndrome. Chin Med J 2013;126: 3245–50.

37. Rey de Castro J, Rosales-Mayor E. Clinical and polysomnographic differences between OSAH patients with/without excessive daytime sleepiness. Sleep Breath 2013;17:1079–86.

38. Jacobsen JH, Shi L, Mokhlesi B. Factors associated with excessive daytime sleepiness in patients with severe obstructive sleep apnea. Sleep Breath 2013;17:629–35.

39. Ryu HS, Lee SA, Lee GH, et al. Subjective apnea symptoms are associated with daytime sleepiness in patients with moderate and severe obstructive

sleep apnoea: a retrospective study. Clin Otolar-yngol 2016;41:395–401.

40. Li Y, Vgontzas AN, Fernandez-Mendoza J, et al. Objective, but not subjective, sleepiness is associated with inflammation in sleep apnea. Sleep 2017; 40(2). https://doi.org/10.1093/sleep/zsw033.

41. Prasad B, Steffen AD, Van Dongen HPA, et al. Determinants of sleepiness in obstructive sleep apnea. Sleep 2018. https://doi.org/10.1093/sleep/zsx199.

42. Barceló A, Barbé F, de la Peña M, et al. Insulin resistance and daytime sleepiness in patients with sleep apnoea. Thorax 2008;63:946–50.

43. Sánchez-de-la-Torre M, Barceló A, Piérola J, et al. Plasma levels of neuropeptides and metabolic hormones, and sleepiness in obstructive sleep apnoea. Respir Med 2011;105:1954–60.

44. Pamidi S, Knutson KL, Ghods F, et al. Depressive symptoms and obesity as predictors of sleepiness and quality of life in patients with REM-related obstructive sleep apnea: cross-sectional analysis of a large clinical population. Sleep Med 2011;12: 827–31.

45. Bonsignore MR, Esquinas C, Barceló A, et al. Metabolic syndrome, insulin resistance and sleepiness in real-life obstructive sleep apnoea. Eur Respir J 2012;39:1136–43.

46. Slater G, Pengo MF, Kosky C, et al. Obesity as an independent predictor of subjective excessive daytime sleepiness. Respir Med 2013;107:305–9.

47. Uysal A, Liendo C, McCarty DE, et al. Nocturnal hypoxemia biomarker predicts sleepiness in patients with severe obstructive sleep apnea. Sleep Breath 2014;18:77–84.

48. Huamaní C, Rey de Castro J, Mezones-Holguin E. Sleepiness and nocturnal hypoxemia in Peruvian men with obstructive sleep apnea. Sleep Breath 2014;18:467–73.

49. Corlateanu A, Pylchenko S, Sircu V, et al. Predictors of daytime sleepiness in patients with obstructive sleep apnea. Pneumologia 2015;64:21–5.

50. Johns MW. A new method for measuring daytime sleepiness: the Epworth sleepiness scale. Sleep 1991;14:540–5.

51. Bonnet MH. ACNS clinical controversy: MSLT and MWT have limited clinical utility. J Clin Neurophysiol 2006;23:50–8.

52. Arzi L, Shreter R, El-Ad B, et al. Forty- versus 20-minute trials of the Maintenance of Wakefulness Test regimen for licensing of drivers. J Clin Sleep Med 2009;5:57–62.

53. Vgontzas AN, Bixler EO, Tan TL, et al. Obesity without sleep apnea is associated with daytime sleepiness. Arch Intern Med 1998;158:1333–7.

54. Resta O, Foschino Barbaro MP, Bonfitto P, et al. Low sleep quality and daytime sleepiness in obese patients without obstructive sleep apnoea syndrome. J Intern Med 2003;253:536–43.

55. Connor J, Norton R, Ameratunga S, et al. Driver sleepiness and risk of serious injury to car occupants: population based case control study. BMJ 2002;324:1125.

56. Horne JA, Reyner LA. Sleep related vehicle accidents. BMJ 1995;310:565–7.

57. Philip P, Vervialle F, Le Breton P, et al. Fatigue, alcohol, and serious road crashes in France: factorial study of national data. BMJ 2001;322:829–30.

58. Sagaspe P, Taillard J, Bayon V, et al. Sleepiness, near-misses and driving accidents among a representative population of French drivers. J Sleep Res 2010;19:578–84.

59. Tefft BC. Prevalence of motor vehicle crashes involving drowsy drivers, United States, 199-2008. Accid Anal Prev 2012;45:180–6.

60. Bioulac S, Micoulaud-Franchi's JA, Arnoud M, et al. Risk of motor vehicle accidents related to sleepiness at the wheel: a systematic review and meta-analysis. Sleep 2017;40(10). https://doi.org/10.1093/sleep/zsx134.

61. Ohayon MM. Determining the level of sleepiness in the American population and its correlates. J Psychiatr Res 2012;46:422–7.

62. Horne J, Reyner L. Vehicle accidents related to sleep: a review. Occup Environ Med 1999;56: 289–94.

63. Garbarino S, Nobili L, Beelke M, et al. The contributing role of sleepiness in highway vehicle accidents. Sleep 2001;24:203–6.

64. Dinges DF. An overview of sleepiness and accidents. J Sleep Res 1995;4(S2):4–14.

65. American Academy of Sleep Medicine. International classification of sleep disorders. 3nd edition. Darien (IL): American Academy of Sleep Medicine; 2014.

66. Herrmann US, Hess CW, Guggisberg AG, et al. Sleepiness is not always perceived before falling asleep in healthy, sleep-deprived subjects. Sleep Med 2010;11:747–51.

67. Verster JC, Mooren L, Bervoets AC, et al. Highway driving safety the day after using sleep medication: the direction of lapses and excursion out-of-lane in drowsy car. J Sleep Res 2018;27:1–4.

68. Dement WC, Carskadon MA. Current perspectives on daytime sleepiness: the issues. Sleep 1982; 5(Suppl 2):S56–66.

69. Masa JF, Rubio M, Findley LJ, et al. Habitually sleepy drivers have a high frequency of automobile crashes associated with respiratory disorders during sleep. Am J Respir Crit Care Med 2000;162: 1407–12.

70. Goncalves M, Amici R, Lucas R, et al. Sleepiness at the wheel across Europe: a survey of 19 countries. J Sleep Res 2015;24:242–53.

71. Maia Q, Grandner MA, Findley J, et al. Short and long sleep duration and risk of drowsy driving and the role of subjective sleep insufficiency. Accid Anal Prev 2013;59:618–22.

72. Anund A, Kecklund G, Kircher A, et al. The effects of driving situation on sleepiness indicators after sleep loss: a driving simulator study. Ind Health 2009;47: 393–401.

73. Filtness AJ, Reyer LA, Horne JA. Driver sleepiness-comparison between young and older men during a monotonous afternoon simulated drive. Biol Psychol 2012;89:580–3.

74. Miyata S, Noda A, Ozaki N, et al. Insufficient sleep impairs driving performance and cognitive function. Neurosci Lett 2010;469:229–33.

75. Sandberg D, Anund A, Fors C, et al. The characteristics of sleepiness during real driving at night–a study of driving performance, physiology and subjective experience. Sleep 2011;34:1317–25.

76. Sunwoo JS, Hwangbo Y, Kim WJ, et al. Sleep characteristics associated with drowsy driving. Sleep Med 2017;40:4–10.

77. Van Dongen HPA, Baynard MD, Dinges DF. Systematic interindividual differences in neurobehavioral impairment from sleep loss: evidence of trait-like differential vulnerability. Sleep 2004;27:423–33.

78. Ahlstrom C, Anund A, Fors C, et al. The effect of daylight versus darkness on driver sleepiness: a driving simulator study. J Sleep Res 2018;27:1–9.

79. Tefft BC. Acute sleep deprivation and culpable motor vehicle crash involvement. Sleep 2018;41:1–11.

80. Ellen RL, Marshall SC, Palayew M, et al. Systematic review of motor vehicle crash risk in persons with sleep apnea. J Clin Sleep Med 2006;15:193–200.

81. Tregear S, Reston J, Schoelles K, et al. Obstructive sleep apnea and risk of motor vehicle crash: systematic review and meta-analysis. J Clin Sleep Med 2009;5:573–81.

82. Garbarino S, Guglielmi O, Sanna A, et al. Risk of occupational accidents in workers with obstructive sleep apnea: systematic review and meta-analysis. Sleep 2016;39:1211–8.

83. Rajaratnam SM, Barger LK, Lockley SW, et al. Sleep disorders, health, and safety in police officers. JAMA 2011;306:2567–78.

84. Karimi M, Hedner J, Habek H, et al. Sleep apnea related risk of motor vehicle accidents is reduced by continuous positive airway pressure: Swedish traffic accident registry data. Sleep 2015;38:341–9.

85. Karimi M, Hedner J, Lombardi C, et al. Driving habits and risk factors fort traffic accidents among sleep apnea patients – a European multi-centre cohort study. J Sleep Res 2014;23:689–99.

86. Garbarino S, Pitidis A, Giustini M, et al. Motor vehicle accidents and obstructive sleep apnea syndrome: a methodology to calculate the related burden of injuries. Chron Respir Dis 2015;12:320–8.

87. Sassani A, Findley LJ, Kryger M, et al. Reducing motor-vehicle collisions, costs, and fatalities by treating obstructive sleep apnea syndrome. Sleep 2004;27:453–8.

88. Tregear S, Reston J, Schoelles K, et al. Continuous positive airway pressure reduces risk of motor vehicle crash among drivers with obstructive sleep apnea. Sleep 2010;33:1373–80.

89. Antonopoulos CN, Sergentanis TN, Daskalopoulou SS, et al. Nasal continuous positive airway pressure (nCPAP) treatment for obstructive sleep apnea, road traffic accidents and driving simulator performance: a meta-analysis. Sleep Med Rev 2011;15:301–10.

90. Burks SV, Anderson JE, Bombyk M, et al. Nonadherence with employer-mandated sleep apnea treatment and increased risk of serious truck crashes. Sleep 2016;39:967–75.

91. Garbarino S, Durando P, Guglielmi O, et al. Sleep apnea, sleep debt and daytime sleepiness are independently associated with road accidents. A cross-sectional study on truck drivers. PLoS One 2016;11: e0166262.

92. Gurubhagavatula I, Sullivan S, Meoli A, et al. Management of obstructive sleep apnea in commercial motor vehicle operators: recommendations of the AASM Sleep and Transportation Safety Awareness Task Force. J Clin Sleep Med 2017;13:745–58.

93. Commission Directive 2014/85/EU of July 1st, 2014, amending Directive 2006/126/EC of the European Parliament and of the Council on driving licenses. Official Journal of the EU, 2.7.2014.

94. Bonsignore MR, Randerath W, Riha R, et al. New rules on driver licensing for patients with obstructive sleep apnoea: EU Directive 2014/85/EU. Eur Respir J 2016;47(1):39–41.

95. Dwarakanath A, Twiddy M, Ghosh D, et al. Variability in clinicians' opinions regarding fitness to drive in patients with obstructive sleep apnoea syndrome (OSAS). Thorax 2015;70:495–7.

96. Phillips CL, Grunstein RR, Darendeliler MA, et al. Health outcomes of continuous positive airway pressure versus oral appliance treatment for obstructive sleep apnea: a randomized controlled trial. Am J Respir Crit Care Med 2013;187:879–87.

97. Rabelo Guimarães Mde L, Hermont AP. Sleep apnea and occupational accidents: are oral appliances the solution? Indian J Occup Environ Med 2014;18: 39–47.

Assessment of Sleepiness in Drivers
Current Methodology and Future Possibilities

Akshay Dwarakanath, MD, MRCP (Respiratory Medicine), FRCP (Edin)[a],
Mark W. Elliott, MD, FERS[b],*

KEYWORDS

- Subjective sleepiness • Objective sleepiness • Driving simulators • Road traffic accidents
- Fitness to drive

KEY POINTS

- There is a strong association between obstructive sleep apnea syndrome and road traffic accidents, with sleepiness being the key factor increasing the risk of an accident.
- Subjective and objective tests of sleepiness have limitations, particularly in the context of assessing the risk of an individual having an accident while driving.
- Advanced driving simulators hold promise, but still remain a research tool.

INTRODUCTION

According to the World Health Organization (WHO), road traffic accidents (RTAs) were the eighth leading cause of death for people of all ages in 2016 and led to 1.35 million injuries worldwide.[1] Death rates are 3 times higher in low-income than in high-income countries. For every death on Europe's roads, there are an estimated 4 permanently disabling injuries, such as damage to the brain or spinal cord, 8 serious injuries, and 50 minor injuries.[2] RTAs are expensive, with each fatal accident costing more than £1 million.[3]

Driving a vehicle is a skill that requires complex integrated higher cortical function, alertness, concentration, and eye to hand coordination.[4] An RTA can be caused by human error, environmental issues such as bad weather, poor road maintenance, or mechanical issues with the vehicle. Up to one-fifth (20%) of accidents on motorways and other monotonous types of roads may be caused by driver fatigue and sleepiness.[5] Sleepiness is the greatest single risk factor for an RTA.[6] The morbidity and mortality associated with a sleep-related RTA are high, caused by greater speed on impact and no, or poor, reaction to an impending event.[5,7] RTAs related to sleepiness are more common in individuals driving alone or for a long distance without a break, in shift workers, and in those with untreated sleep disorders.[7] A sleep-related RTA can also occur during circadian rhythm changes, when vigilance is low (afternoon and nights); driving under the influence

Disclosure: A. Dwarakanath reports travel expenses and fees for speaking from Respironics. M.W. Elliott reports honoraria, travel expenses, and subsistence from Resmed, Philips Respironics, and Fisher and Paykel.
[a] Department of Respiratory Medicine, Sleep and Non-invasive Ventilation Service, Mid Yorkshire Hospitals NHS Trust, Aberford Road, Wakefield, West Yorkshire WF2 9EU, UK; [b] Department of Respiratory Medicine, Sleep and Non-invasive Ventilation Service, St. James's University Hospital, Beckett Street, Leeds, West Yorkshire LS9 7TF, UK
* Corresponding author.
E-mail address: mwelliott@doctors.org.uk

Sleep Med Clin 14 (2019) 441–451
https://doi.org/10.1016/j.jsmc.2019.08.003

of alcohol or medications; in sleep deprivation; and in shift workers.[8] Two-thirds of drivers who fall asleep at the wheel are car drivers, 85% of the drivers causing sleep-related RTAs are men, and more than one-third are less than 30 years of age.[9]

Poor sleep hygiene is the commonest cause of excessive daytime sleepiness (EDS), and untreated obstructive sleep apnea syndrome (OSAS) is the most common medical condition causing EDS.[10] A meta-analysis comparing the risks for RTA in all medical conditions reported that OSAS has an increased risk, between 1.2-fold and 2-fold, with respect to a healthy population. It has the highest increased risk, which is second only to age and sex as a general risk factor for RTA.[11] However, these studies of OSAS as a risk factor for RTA (**Table 1**) had limitations; small numbers, unmatched controls, possible underreporting (being based on self-reported accidents rather than an objective record from police or licensing authorities), a lack of robust questionnaire data, issues about recall and gender bias, and no data on the severity of the sleep disordered breathing.

Although sleepiness is likely to be the main factor explaining increased accident rates in OSAS, there are other possible factors to be considered. OSAS is associated with focal loss of gray matter; subtle cerebellar damage, affecting coordination, in particular may have an impact on an individual's driving abilities.[19] Tippin and colleagues[20] reported that drivers with OSAS have reduced visual vigilance for peripheral targets and postulated that this effect is caused by a decline in attention and fatigue. Obesity may influence mechanical aspects of driving and increased body mass index has been shown to be an independent predictor of accident risk in some studies. Alcohol or drugs reduce reaction times and lead to poor decision making, which may add to accident risk; Terán-Santos and colleagues[16] showed that people with OSAS who had consumed any alcohol were at increased risk of being involved in an RTA compared with those who had consumed no alcohol before an RTA.

Driving is an essential part of modern life and most patients with OSAS drive motor vehicles. A survey by the British Lung Foundation (BLF) showed that, among a cohort of patients with OSAS (n = 2671) attending sleep clinics in the United Kingdom, 82% of responders held a current driving license, 62% drove a motor vehicle, and 16% held a professional driving license or drove for a living.[21] Making a decision about whether an individual is fit to drive is therefore an important issue in this patient group.

Commercial drivers represent a particular challenge to the sleep community. There is good evidence that sleepiness, irrespective of the cause, is a major risk factor for both RTAs and other accidents at work.[22–25] Rates of sleepiness and sleep-related accidents among professional drivers are high[26] because of a combination of factors, including shift work. Accidents involving commercial drivers may be particularly harmful because they operate large vehicles, transport hazardous materials, carry multiple passengers, operate for long stretches of time, and may have an economic incentive to continue driving when noncommercial drivers may choose to stop. Multiple risk factors may synergistically increase the risk of accidents.[27]

Sagaspe and colleagues[23] undertook telephone interviews with both commercial and noncommercial drivers in France and found that 11.8% had an Epworth Sleepiness Score (ESS) greater than 11; 28.6% reported sleepiness at the wheel severe enough to require stopping, 46.8% felt sleepy during nighttime driving and 39.4% during daytime driving, 10% had had a near miss during the previous year, and 6% had had a driving accident. Howard and colleagues[28] showed that 60% of commercial drivers had sleep disordered breathing and 24% were excessively sleepy. A survey conducted in Norway found that 63% of cargo drivers, 52% of passenger train operators, 29% of maritime watch officers, and 26% of bus and

Table 1
The risk of road traffic accident in obstructive sleep apnea syndrome

Author, Year	Type of Study	Risk of RTA in OSAS
Findley et al,[12] 1988	Case control (n = 29/35)	OR, 7.0
Haraldsson et al,[13] 1990	Case control (n = 140/142)	OR, 12.0
Young et al,[14] 1997	General population (n = 913)	OR, 3.4
George & Smiley,[15] 1999	Case control (n = 460/581)	OR, 2.0
Terán-Santos et al,[16] 1999	Case control (n = 102/152)	OR, 6.3 if AHI>10/h
Horstmann et al,[17] 2000	Case control (n = 156/160)	OR, 12.0
Mulgrew et al,[18] 2008	Case control (n = 783/783)	Severe OSAS, RR 2.0

Abbreviations: AHI, apnea-hypopnea index; OR, odds ratio; RR, relative risk.

truck drivers admitted to nodding off or slept at least once while driving in the 3 months preceding the survey.[29] In sleep questionnaire data obtained from 677 drivers employed at bus depots in Edinburgh, United Kingdom, 20% reported an ESS greater than 10, 8% reported falling asleep at the wheel at least once a month, 7% reported having had an accident, and 18% reported having had a near-miss accident because of sleepiness while working.[26] A survey of heavy goods vehicle drivers reported an average accident liability of 0.26 accidents in a 3-year recall period; accident liability increased with increasing ESS scores.[30] A systematic review and meta-analysis by Garbarino and colleagues[31] showed that, compared with controls, the odds of an accident at work were nearly double in workers with OSAS (odds ratio [OR], 2.18; 95% confidence interval [CI], 1.53–3.10). One problem with most of these studies is that patients, particularly when it has implications for their employment, may be reluctant to report accidents and may underreport symptoms.[32] However, data from police, relevant licensing authorities, and insurers also tend to underestimate the issue because not all incidents are reported, particularly near misses caused by nodding episodes that have not resulted in an accident.

POSITION STATEMENTS ABOUT OBSTRUCTIVE SLEEP APNEA SYNDROME AND DRIVING

The increased risk of RTA has prompted a consideration of OSAS in the framework of legislation for driving licenses. Rules for medical assessment before obtaining a driving license differ from country to country. Position statements in recent years by various medical bodies[33,34] and licensing authorities[35] have attempted to tackle this issue. The American Thoracic Society (ATS) clinical practice guideline on sleep apnea, sleepiness, and driving risk in noncommercial drivers[34] considers patients to be high-risk drivers if there is moderate to severe sleepiness and a recent unintended RTA or near miss attributable to sleepiness, fatigue, or inattention. It states that there is no compelling evidence to restrict driving privileges in patients with OSAS if there has not been such an episode.

Annexe iii of the European Union (EU) directive on driving licenses was revised in 2014 on the recommendations from a working group established by the Transport and Mobility Directorate of the European Commission in 2012.[36] The directive, which was subject to mandatory implementation by all member states from December 2015, states that, "Applicants or drivers in whom a moderate or severe OSAS is suspected shall be referred to

further authorised medical advice before a driving licence is issued or renewed."[36] They may be advised not to drive until confirmation of the diagnosis. Driving licenses may be issued to applicants or drivers with moderate or severe OSAS who show adequate control of their condition and compliance with appropriate treatment and improvement of sleepiness, if any, confirmed by authorized medical opinion. Applicants or drivers with moderate or severe OSAS under treatment shall be subject to a periodic medical review, at intervals not exceeding 3 years for drivers of group 1 (ie, noncommercial drivers) and 1 year for drivers of group 2 (ie, commercial drivers), with a view to establishing the level of compliance with treatment, the need for continuing the treatment, and continued good vigilance.[36] The European Respiratory Society has established a task force to develop guidance and help ensure that any adoption of EU 2014/85/EU is undertaken in a reasoned, sustainable, and fair manner in line with each country's legislative procedures and economic resources.[37,38]

At present in the United Kingdom, the Driving Vehicle Licensing Authority (DVLA)[35] has guidelines that are applicable to all drivers who have OSAS. The DVLA has focused on sleepiness sufficient to impair driving along and severity of sleep apnea based on apnea-hypopnea index (AHI) or equivalent. Patients should inform the DVLA and complete the relevant form (SL1 for class 1 and SLV1 for class 2 licenses) after a diagnosis of OSAS has been confirmed. Once the DVLA is informed, medical enquiries are undertaken to establish whether the driver should retain the license. The DVLA remains the final arbiter, but their guidance is based on information from the individual driver and the treating clinician. Driving is normally allowed to continue once satisfactory control of the condition is achieved, and this should be confirmed by the clinician. Not reporting a diagnosis of OSAS to the DVLA could result in a £1000 fine. Whatever is decided, it is still the patient's responsibility not to drive on any occasion if feeling sleepy. Individuals may be safe to drive almost all of the time, but not safe just on 1 occasion when they have been temporarily sleep deprived for whatever reason.

ASSESSMENT OF SLEEPINESS AND DRIVING RISK

Clinicians are often asked to make recommendations about fitness to drive, which can be challenging, with major implications for the patient's livelihood, in particular for professional drivers. There is a duty of care on clinicians to discourage patients who are at high risk of causing an accident from driving or even to report them to the licensing authorities. The UK General Medical Council (GMC) has published guidance about breaching patient confidentiality in certain extreme circumstances in the interests of public safety.[39] Patients with OSAS have to obey the law, but, because of the fear of losing their driving license or livelihood, may under-report sleepiness at the wheel. A meta-analysis showed that making patients take the issue of potential unsafe driving seriously using threats generates fear and does not translate into positive change resulting in less risky driving behavior.[40] Clinicians' warnings to patients who are potentially unfit to drive may contribute to a decrease in subsequent RTAs but may also exacerbate mood disorders and compromise the doctor-patient relationship.[41] They may also dissuade others from seeking treatment of their own symptoms. Ideally, the patient and clinician should agree that any decision taken is reasonable and can be justified, but sometimes it is impossible to avoid conflict. A British Thoracic Society survey showed that the advice given by a clinician is inconsistent not only at the time of diagnosis but also following treatment with CPAP.[42] There are discordant views regarding residual sleepiness and adequate CPAP compliance.[42] Such variation shows that clinicians require more guidance in the assessment of driving in patients with OSAS. Objective tests should bring standardization and greater consistency, but no such test currently exists. This article considers several potential options.

Assessment of Sleepiness: Subjective

Sleepiness varies over time. What constitutes normal alertness, particularly during driving, is poorly defined. The relationship between sleepiness in general and RTAs is not consistent. Terán-Santos and colleagues[16] did not find any relationship, but a Chinese study reported a higher chance of RTAs (OR, 2.07) in people with chronic sleepiness when assessed by ESS (>10).[43]

Different validated subjective scales have been used to assess self-reported sleepiness in both clinical and research settings. The ESS,[44] a well-validated questionnaire, is the most commonly used scoring system to assess EDS in OSAS. It was introduced in 1991 by Dr Murray Johns of Epworth Hospital in Melbourne, Australia. It is easy to administer and is useful in measuring changes in sleepiness over time. It measures daytime sleepiness on a probability scale of 0 to 3 in 8 different situations during the day. It has a total score of 24 and a score of less than 10 is

considered normal. There are various limitations to the ESS. A study in older adults concluded that most older adults were not able to answer all of the ESS items and the ESS may underestimate sleepiness severity in older people.[45] Close relative–evaluated ESS performs as well as, if not better than, self-evaluated ESS and may be useful in some situations.[46] People may underplay their responses, leading to bias, particularly when they think driving risk might be being assessed. The Stanford Sleepiness Score uses a 7-point scale (1, fully alert; 7, struggling to stay awake) and the immediate state of sleepiness is assessed. It is a subjective assessment of an individual's alertness. However, there is no relation to the severity of OSAS and it is used only before Multiple Sleep Latency Test (MSLT).[47] It is not useful for assessing the propensity for sleepiness during driving. Guaita and colleagues[48] recently developed the Barcelona Sleepiness Index, which is a questionnaire of just 2 items, which correlates well with objective sleepiness measures and oxyhemoglobin desaturation, and is sensitive to change with therapy.

With regard to accident risk, the key issue is whether patients experience sleepiness while driving. Masa and colleagues[49] suggested that asking about EDS while driving, rather than sleepiness in general, may better predict which subjects with OSAS are at risk of RTAs.

All subjective measures of sleepiness rely on the insight and honesty of the patients (or their close relatives) and this is a major limitation of all scores based on patient self-report. Careful observation of the manner and body language of the patient and partner during the consultation can help to identify likely inconsistencies, and, when these are identified, issues should be explored carefully and sensitively. Responses can be challenged; for example, a patient with a low ESS who was asleep in the waiting room or in whom answers to other questions about inappropriate sleepiness suggest a much bigger problem than that suggested by an, inappropriately, low ESS. The converse is also true; the Epworth test asks about the likelihood of falling asleep in various situations, not whether patients actually do so. Furthermore, one person's high chance is another's moderate chance. The patient's attitude/reaction to a near miss while driving is also important. Individuals who have adapted their driving behavior in response to an episode are likely to be at less risk of a future accident than individuals who does not seem to appreciate the significance and carry on regardless. Although clinician experience is likely to be helpful in evaluating sleepiness and its likely impact on safe driving, it will always be a difficult area.

Assessment of Sleepiness: Objective Tests

There are several objective tests of sleepiness, measuring different aspects of sleepiness. The MSLT,[50] Maintenance of Wakefulness Test (MWT),[51] and Oxford Sleep Resistance (OSLER) test[52] are useful clinical tests for the evaluation of excessive sleepiness but all have limitations, particularly with respect to assessing the impact of sleepiness on driving. The MSLT assesses an individual's ability to fall asleep during the day and, intuitively, it is not appropriate to assess a patient's fitness to drive because patients do not try to fall asleep while driving.[53] Young and colleagues[14] found no difference in MSLT test scores between subjects involved in an RTA and those who were not.

The MWT is more logical. This test is a validated and objective measure of the ability of an individual to stay awake, which is more reflective of is done when driving (ie, trying to maintain alertness). It is of some use in evaluating the driving performance in sleepy patients.[54–58] The same is true of the OSLER, a behavioral equivalent of the MWT.[52] There is a relationship between driving ability and the MWT in patients with untreated obstructive sleep apnea.[54,55] Pathologic sleep latencies on the MWT predict simulator driving impairment in patients with hypersomnias of central origin, as well as in patients with OSAS.[58] A pathologic MWT is associated with simulated driving impairment; sleepy patients had more inappropriate line crossings than control drivers ($P<.05$),[55] but its suitability to evaluate real-world performances and/or risks has been questioned.[56–58] It is not sufficiently discriminating for everyday practice. Furthermore, patients can reasonably question a decision to disallow driving based on an abnormal MWT, arguing that, when driving, they are stimulated and concentrating, which is not the case when performing the MWT (or OSLER test). In addition, these tests of sleepiness do not test any other aspects of driver performance that may affect safety.

Driving Simulators

Intuitively, a driving simulator is the most logical test, because it potentially can test factors other than sleepiness that are important for safe driving. It is also more credible for patients. There are a variety of different approaches to simulating driving.

A hierarchy can be considered:

1. The steer-clear test. It is marginal as to whether this should be considered a driving simulator, but it has been used in various studies as a measure of driving performance. A vehicle is shown on a screen moving on a 2-lane highway. Obstacles (steers) intermittently appear in the vehicle's lane. To avoid hitting an obstacle, the subject has to move the vehicle to the other lane by pressing the space bar on the keyboard, thereby measuring reaction time.[59–65]

2. Divided-attention steering simulators (DASSs). A computer-based image of the moving edges of a winding road are portrayed by lines on a computer screen. A rudimentary image of the bonnet of the vehicle is displayed at the bottom of the screen. Using a standard computer game steering wheel, the subject steers the center of the vehicle as accurately as possible down the center of the road. Deviation from this is recorded as tracking error. Single digits, which randomly change, are displayed at each corner of the computer screen and each time a target digit appears (approximately once per minute), the subject presses a button on either side of the steering wheel. By including this visual search task, a divided-attention task is produced.[54,65–75]

3. Personal computer (PC)–based simulators with more realistic graphics, driving environment, and vehicle controls.[76–88] The subject is expected to drive the road normally, usually following a lead vehicle and sometimes needing to respond to a programmed event, which tests reaction time and so forth. A variety of parameters can be measured continuously (discussed later).

4. Fully immersive simulators.[20,58,83,89–91] The driving experience realistically replicates that of real driving, with complex audiovisuals and the feeling of the car responding to the controls and so forth, but such simulators are expensive to build and run. They provide a close to real-life driving experience and multiple parameters can be measured easily, either from the car controls (eg, accuracy of steering, speed variation, braking reaction time) or from additional monitoring equipment (electroencephalogram, eye camera). The subject can be required to react to situations or perform other tasks and so forth that on a real road could cause an accident, in complete safety.

5. Real-life on-road driving[73] in an instrumented car with the ability to measure multiple parameters both in the driver and the car. This test is the gold standard but is limited by cost and availability. Safety considerations may also be

an issue; undertaking such studies is unethical if the individual is considered to be at high risk of having an accident.

Some studies have evaluated different components of driving in separate neuropsychiatric tests rather than integrated into a simulator or in addition to a simulator.[61,92,93]

The more realistic the simulator, the fewer the events, both in patients and normal people. During test drives on simple simulators, the number of off-road events, crashes, and so forth during a short run is much higher than would be expected in the same individual during real driving. For example, in one study,[72] although patients had more off-road events than general subjects, both still had unacceptably high instances (90 ± 71 vs 40 ± 36 per hour), which is not reflective of real-world normal driving. By contrast, Ghosh and colleagues,[86] using a PC-based simulator with more realistic graphics, showed that more than 50% of patients with OSAS of sufficient severity to warrant a trial of CPAP could complete approximately 1 hour of motorway driving without deviating out of the assigned lane, crashing and so forth. This observation has been made in other studies using more sophisticated simulators. When driving performance is evaluated through quantitative performance measures (eg, standard deviation of lane position [SDLP]), simulated driving is generally seen to be worse, with higher absolute values compared with real-road test driving.[91] The more realistic the driving experience, the greater the cost, which has implications for a clinical test.

The most commonly evaluated end points on a simulator include crashes, near misses, drifting out of lane (inappropriate line crossings), how well the individual maintains position on the road (tracking error, SDLP, lane position in centimeters), reaction time, and speed adjustment. SDLP most consistently correlates with sleepiness and performance on the simulator.[86,94] Patients with OSAS perform worse than normal people on driving simulators of all types.[20,58,59,61,62,64,66–68,70,72,74,76,80,82,85,88,89,92,95,96] This finding holds true for crashes, drifting out of lane/inappropriate line crossing, and continuously measured variables. Performance on simulators is worse in situations in which real driving performance is expected to be worse (eg, after alcohol or sleep deprivation[78,82,83,95]) and improves following treatment of the sleep disordered breathing.[63,64,68,69,83,85,89,93,97,98] Simulated driving is worse in sleepy patients.[54,58,75,79,81,84] Several studies[65,71,86] have shown that women perform worse than men on simulators, which is surprising because women generally experience fewer accidents during real-world driving than men. Furthermore, women are more often involved in low-speed accidents involving visual-spatial skills (eg, parking) than higher-speed accidents. It is the latter type of driving that is generally tested on simulators.

Most studies use a driving simulator to help understand mechanisms by which OSAS might compromise safe driving, as a comparator with other tests that measure aspects of OSAS likely to compromise safe driving (eg, sleepiness as measured by MSLT or MWT) or as an end point to indicate effective treatment. Few studies compared simulated driving with real-life events. However in those that did, there were relationships, albeit weak, with self-reported sleepiness in general (ESS), accidents, episodes of drowsing, or sleepiness at the wheel.[60,65,71,87,91] These relationships were seen with steer-clear,[60,65] DASS,[71] and more sophisticated PC-based simulators.[87,91] However, such a relationship has not been seen in other studies.[61] Studies involving the most realistic simulators involved too few subjects for meaningful comparison with real-life events.

Based on the current evidence, driving simulators are not able to predict reliably real-life near misses or accidents at an individual level. This inability is not surprising; individuals who have crashes in real cars caused by sleepiness are very likely to have been driving the same car on many previous occasions without incident. That a driver crashes on 1 occasion during simulated driving but not on another is consistent with what happens during real, everyday driving. Accidents are also caused by other drivers and by factors other than driver sleepiness; for example, mechanical failure, poor roads, and adverse weather conditions. Measures, such as SDLP, that are measured continuously or reaction time may be more useful. Abnormal values may indicate individuals who are close to the threshold for having an accident, even if, to date, they have not had one. It can be likened to individuals walking along a cliff edge; they may not have fallen over yet, but they are at more risk than someone who is walking further away from the edge.

Poor performance on a driving simulator alone should not be used to prevent an individual from driving; however, given the consistent relationship with sleepiness in many studies, poor performance should at least raise a question about whether that individual is safe to drive.

CURRENT STATUS

The determination of driver future accident risk requires a multifaceted approach by an experienced clinician. Several factors need to be considered.

There is a weak relationship between the severity of the sleep disordered breathing and the risk of RTAs,[17,99,100] and patients should not be prevented from driving because of the presence of sleep disordered breathing alone. The same is true for sleep disordered breathing plus symptoms (ie, OSAS). Clinicians assessing patients with OSAS should ask specific questions regarding driving behavior; previous accidents, near-miss events, or a history of recurrent nodding in the last 12 months should be considered red flags and individuals should be advised to refrain from driving. There is synergistic increase in risk when 2 or more risk factors occur in the same individual.[27] Other factors may increase the risk for drowsy driving, such as medication (eg, sedatives), substance use (eg, alcohol), and other sleep problems (eg, sleep restriction), and medical comorbidities should be considered in the decision-making process. Despite their limitations, in the absence of better tests, the objective tests described earlier have a role, but, given the lack of evidence, results must not be given undue weight.

FUTURE POSSIBILITIES

Any test to assess driving accident risk should fulfill several criteria (**Box 1**). More complex driving simulators potentially do this, but future research should focus on standardization of simulator outcomes, determining which of the many outputs available from a simulator are the best predictors of real-life events, and the optimal length of the test. There needs to be a consistent definition of accidents and near misses, attributable to driver fatigue. Continuous measures that indicate that the driver is at increased risk of a fatigue-related accident (eg, position variation within the lane) currently seem to be the most useful measures, but further work is required to delineate the relationship with

real-life accidents and whether the measure is repeatable over time and sensitive to change. Further work on the usefulness, or otherwise, is required in women. Modern cars incorporate technologies to alert the driver to fatigue, but none of these have been robustly validated to reduce accidents. However, they are likely to be helpful unless they lead drivers to rely on them inappropriately and continue to drive when they should have stopped for a rest. Research continues apace into the use of artificial intelligence and driverless cars, and if (when) they become mainstream, all of the earlier discussion will be redundant.

SUMMARY

In common with many other situations in clinical practice, a decision about whether an individual should cease driving is complex and cannot be based on simple yes-or-no criteria. This article suggests a multifaceted approach that should include a summative assessment of severity of sleepiness, each element of which needs to be weighed for significance. Advanced driving simulators hold promise and offer potential practical value because simulated driving in sleepy individuals is partially related to their real driving performance. Importance should be given to self-perception of sleepiness-related impairment and risky behavior. Licensing authorities remain the final arbiters of which individuals should cease driving, but they should be guided by clinicians. Individuals should be advised of their personal responsibility; they may be safe to drive most of the time, but not after a poor night's sleep. No one should drive on any occasion if they cannot guarantee to maintain full concentration and vigilance; this applies to all drivers, not just those with OSAS.

Box 1
Requirements for tests on which decisions are to be made about driving

- Should be practical
- Should be credible
- Should have some relationship with accident history (this need not be a strong relationship)
- Should be reproducible
- Ideally the subject should not be aware of what is being measured
- Should be measured continuously

REFERENCES

1. Global status report on road safety 2018. Available at: https://www.who.int/violence_injury_prevention/road_safety_status/2018/en/. Accessed September 15, 2019.
2. European Commission. Road safety. Statistics-accidents data. 2019. Available at: http://ec.europa.eu/transport/road_safety/specialist/statistics/index_en.htm. Accessed September 15, 2019.
3. Douglas NJ, George CF. Treating sleep apnoea is cost effective. Thorax 2002;57(1):93.
4. Land M, Horwood J. Which parts of the road guide steering? Nature 1995;377(6547):339–40.
5. Horne JA, Reyner LA. Sleep related vehicle accidents. Br Med J 1995;310(6979):565–7.

6. de Mello MT, Narciso FV, Tufik S, et al. Sleep disorders as a cause of motor vehicle collisions. Int J Prev Med 2013;4(3):246–57.

7. Pack AI, Pack AM, Rodgman E, et al. Characteristics of crashes attributed to the driver having fallen asleep. Accid Anal Prev 1995;27(6):769–75.

8. DVLA. Tiredness can kill: advice for drivers (INF159). Available at: www.gov.uk/government/publications/tiredness-can-kill-advice-for-drivers. Accessed September 15, 2019.

9. Fatigue and road safety: a critical analysis of recent evidence" road safety web publication No.21. Department for Transport, Queen's Printer and Controller of Her Majesty's Stationery Office; 2011. Available at: https://webarchive.nationalarchives.gov.uk/20121103213009/http://www.dft.gov.uk/publications/rsrr-theme3-fatigue-road-safety-analysis/. Accessed September 15, 2019.

10. George CF. Sleep apnea, alertness, and motor vehicle crashes. Am J Respir Crit Care Med 2007;176(10):954–6.

11. Vaa T. Summary: impairments diseases, age and their relative risks of accident involvement: results from meta-analysis. Available at: https://www.toi.no/publikasjoner/tilstander-sykdommer-alder-og-relativ-risiko-for-innblanding-i-ulykker-resultater-fra-meta-analyse-article5484-8.html. Accessed September 15, 2019.

12. Findley LJ, Unverzagt ME, Suratt PM. Automobile accidents involving patients with obstructive sleep apnea. Am Rev Respir Dis 1988;138(2):337–40.

13. Haraldsson PO, Carenfelt C, Diderichsen F, et al. Clinical symptoms of sleep apnea syndrome and automobile accidents. ORL J Otorhinolaryngol Relat Spec 1990;52(1):57–62.

14. Young T, Blustein J, Finn L, et al. Sleep-disordered breathing and motor vehicle accidents in a population-based sample of employed adults. Sleep 1997;20:608–13.

15. George CF, Smiley A. Sleep apnea & automobile crashes. Sleep 1999;22(6):790–5.

16. Terán-Santos J, Jimenez-Gomez A, Cordero-Guevara J. The association between sleep apnea and the risk of traffic accidents. Cooperative Group Burgos-Santander. N Engl J Med 1999;340(11):847–51.

17. Horstmann S, Hess CW, Bassetti C, et al. Sleepiness-related accidents in sleep apnea patients. Sleep 2000;23(3):383–9.

18. Mulgrew AT, Nasvadi G, Butt A, et al. Risk and severity of motor vehicle crashes in patients with obstructive sleep apnoea/hypopnoea. Thorax 2008;63(6):536–41.

19. Morrell MJ, Jackson ML, Twigg GL, et al. Changes in brain morphology in patients with obstructive sleep apnoea. Thorax 2010;65(10):908–14.

20. Tippin J, Sparks J, Rizzo M. Visual vigilance in drivers with obstructive sleep apnea. J Psychosom Res 2009;67(2):143–51.

21. Summary report of the BLF's OSA patient experience survey 2014. Available at: https://www.blf.org.uk/file/osa-patient-survey-blf-summary-report-2014. Accessed September 15, 2019.

22. Horne JA, Reyner LA. Driver sleepiness. J Sleep Res 1995;4(S2):23–9.

23. Sagaspe P, Taillard J, Bayon V, et al. Sleepiness, near-misses and driving accidents among a representative population of French drivers. J Sleep Res 2010;19(4):578–84.

24. Garbarino S, Nobili L, Beelke M, et al. The contributing role of sleepiness in highway vehicle accidents. Sleep 2001;24(2):203–6.

25. Garbarino S, Repice AM, Traversa F, et al. Commuting accidents: the influence of excessive daytime sleepiness. A review of an Italian Police officers population. G Ital Med Lav Ergon 2007;29(3 Suppl):324–6 [in Italian].

26. Vennelle M, Engleman HM, Douglas NJ. Sleepiness and sleep-related accidents in commercial bus drivers. Sleep Breath 2010;14(1):39–42.

27. Arndt JT, Wilde GJ, Munt PW, et al. Simulated driving performance following prolonged wakefulness and alcohol consumption: separate and combined contributions to impairment. J Sleep Res 2000;9(3):233–41.

28. Howard ME, Desai AV, Grunstein RR, et al. Sleepiness, sleep-disordered breathing, and accident risk factors in commercial vehicle drivers. Am J Respir Crit Care Med 2004;170(9):1014–21.

29. Phillips RO, Sagberg F, Torkel B. Fatigue in operators of land- and sea-based transport forms in Norway: risk profiles. Fatigue in transport report IV. 2015. Available at: https://www.toi.no/publications/fatigue-in-operators-of-land-and-sea-based-transport-forms-in-norway-risk-profiles-fatigue-in-transport-report-iv-article33571-29.html. Accessed September 15, 2019.

30. Maycock G. Sleepiness and driving: the experience of heavy goods vehicle drivers in the UK. J Sleep Res 1997;6(4):238–44.

31. Garbarino S, Guglielmi O, Sanna A, et al. Risk of occupational accidents in workers with obstructive sleep apnea: systematic review and meta-analysis. Sleep 2016;39(6):1211–8.

32. Engleman HM, Hirst WS, Douglas NJ. Under reporting of sleepiness and driving impairment in patients with sleep apnoea/hypopnoea syndrome. J Sleep Res 1997;6:272–5.

33. British Thoracic Society. Position Statement: driving and obstructive sleep apnoea (OSA)/obstructive sleep apnoea syndrome (OSAS). Available at: https://www.respiratoryfutures.org.uk/news/revised-bts-

position-statement-on-driving-and-osa/. Accessed September 15, 2019.

34. Strohl KP, Brown DB, Collop N, et al. An official American Thoracic Society clinical practice guideline: sleep apnea, sleepiness, and driving risk in noncommercial drivers. An update of a 1994 Statement. Am J Respir Crit Care Med 2013;187(11): 1259–66.

35. Driver and Vehicle Licensing Agency. Miscellaneous conditions: assessing fitness to drive. 2019. Available at: https://assets.publishing.service.gov.uk/government/uploads/system/uploads/attachment_data/file/783444/assessing-fitness-to-drive-a-guide-for-medical-professionals.pdf. Accessed September 15, 2019.

36. McNicholas WT e. New standards and guidelines for drivers with obstructive sleep apnoea syndrome: report of the Obstructive Sleep Apnoea Working Group. Brussels, European Commission. Available at: https://ec.europa.eu/transport/road_safety/sites/roadsafety/files/pdf/behavior/sleep_apnoea.pdf. Accessed September 15, 2019.

37. Bonsignore MR, Randerath W, Riha R, et al. New rules on driver licensing for patients with obstructive sleep apnea: European Union Directive 2014/85/EU. J Sleep Res 2016;25(1):3–4.

38. Bonsignore MR, Randerath W, Riha R, et al. New rules on driver licensing for patients with obstructive sleep apnoea: EU Directive 2014/85/EU. Eur Respir J 2016;47(1):39–41.

39. Confidentiality: patients' fitness to drive and reporting concerns to the DVLA or DVA. 2017. Available at: https://www.gmc-uk.org/ethical-guidance/ethical-guidance-for-doctors/confidentiality—patients-fitness-to-drive-and-reporting-concerns-to-the-dvla-or-dva. Accessed September 15, 2019.

40. Carey RN, McDermott DT, Sarma KM. The impact of threat appeals on fear arousal and driver behavior: a meta-analysis of experimental research 1990-2011. PLoS One 2013;8(5):e62821.

41. Redelmeier DA, Yarnell CJ, Thiruchelvam D, et al. Physicians' warnings for unfit drivers and the risk of trauma from road crashes. N Engl J Med 2012; 367(13):1228–36.

42. Dwarakanath A, Twiddy M, Ghosh D, et al. Variability in clinicians' opinions regarding fitness to drive in patients with obstructive sleep apnoea syndrome (OSAS). Thorax 2015;70(5):495–7.

43. Liu GF, Han S, Liang DH, et al. Driver sleepiness and risk of car crashes in Shenyang, a Chinese northeastern city: population-based case-control study. Biomed Environ Sci 2003;16(3):219–26.

44. Johns MW. Reliability and factor analysis of the Epworth sleepiness scale. Sleep 1992;15:376–81.

45. Onen F, Moreau T, Gooneratne NS, et al. Limits of the Epworth sleepiness scale in older adults. Sleep Breath 2013;17(1):343–50.

46. Li Y, Zhang J, Lei F, et al. Self-evaluated and close relative-evaluated Epworth Sleepiness Scale vs. multiple sleep latency test in patients with obstructive sleep apnea. J Clin Sleep Med 2014;10(2): 171–6.

47. American Academy of Sleep Medicine. International classification of sleep disorders. (3rd edition). Available at: https://learn.aasm.org/Public/Catalog/Details.aspx?id=%2FgqQVDMQIT%2FEDy86PWgqgQ%3D%3D&returnurl=%2FUsers%2FUserOnlineCourse.aspx%3FLearningActivityID%3D%252fgqQVDMQIT%252fEDy86PWgqgQ%253d%253d. Accessed September 15, 2019.

48. Guaita M, Salamero M, Vilaseca I, et al. The Barcelona sleepiness Index: a new instrument to assess excessive daytime sleepiness in sleep disordered breathing. J Clin Sleep Med 2015;11(11):1289–98.

49. Masa JF, Rubio M, Findley LJ. Habitually sleepy drivers have a high frequency of automobile crashes associated with respiratory disorders during sleep. Am J Respir Crit Care Med 2000;162(4 Pt 1):1407–12.

50. Carskadon MA, Dement WC, Mitler MM, et al. Guidelines for the multiple sleep latency test (MSLT): a standard measure of sleepiness. Sleep 1986;9(4):519–24.

51. Littner MR, Kushida C, Wise M, et al. Practice parameters for clinical use of the multiple sleep latency test and the maintenance of wakefulness test. Sleep 2005;28(1):113–21.

52. Bennett LS, Stradling JR, Davies RJ. A behavioural test to assess daytime sleepiness in obstructive sleep apnoea. J Sleep Res 1997;6(2):142–5.

53. Wise MS. Objective measures of sleepiness and wakefulness: application to the real world? J Clin Neurophysiol 2006;23(1):39–49.

54. Sagaspe P, Taillard J, Chaumet G, et al. Maintenance of wakefulness test as a predictor of driving performance in patients with untreated obstructive sleep apnea. Sleep 2007;30(3):327–30.

55. Philip P, Sagaspe P, Taillard J, et al. Maintenance of wakefulness test, obstructive sleep apnea syndrome, and driving risk. Ann Neurol 2008;64(4): 410–6.

56. Bonnet MH. ACNS clinical controversy: MSLT and MWT have limited clinical utility. J Clin Neurophysiol 2006;23(1):50–8.

57. Bonnet MH. The MSLT and MWT should not be used for the assessment of workplace safety. J Clin Sleep Med 2006;2(2):128–31.

58. Philip P, Chaufton C, Taillard J, et al. Maintenance of wakefulness test scores and driving performance in sleep disorder patients and controls. Int J Psychophysiol 2013;89(2):195–202.

59. Findley LJ, Fabrizio MJ, Knight H, et al. Driving simulator performance in patients with sleep apnea. Am Rev Respir Dis 1989;140(2):529–30.

60. Findley L, Unverzagt M, Guchu R, et al. Vigilance and automobile accidents in patients with sleep apnea or narcolepsy. Chest 1995;108:619–24.

61. Barbe, Pericas J, Munoz A, et al. Automobile accidents in patients with sleep apnea syndrome. An epidemiological and mechanistic study. Am J Respir Crit Care Med 1998;158(1):18–22.

62. Findley LJ, Suratt PM, Dinges DF. Time-on-task decrements in "steer clear" performance of patients with sleep apnea and narcolepsy. Sleep 1999; 22(6):804–9.

63. Kingshott RN, Vennelle M, Hoy CJ, et al. Predictors of improvements in daytime function outcomes with CPAP therapy. Am J Respir Crit Care Med 2000; 161(3 Pt 1):866–71.

64. Munoz A, Mayoralas LR, Barbe F, et al. Long-term effects of CPAP on daytime functioning in patients with sleep apnoea syndrome. Eur Respir J 2000; 15(4):676–81.

65. Pichel F, Zamarron C, Magan F, et al. Sustained attention measurements in obstructive sleep apnea and risk of traffic accidents. Respir Med 2006; 100(6):1020–7.

66. George CF, Boudreau AC, Smiley A. Simulated driving performance in patients with obstructive sleep apnea. Am J Respir Crit Care Med 1996; 154:175–81.

67. George CF, Boudreau AC, Smiley A. Comparison of simulated driving performance in narcolepsy and sleep apnea patients. Sleep 1996;19:711–7.

68. George CF, Boudreau AC, Smiley A. Effects of nasal CPAP on simulated driving performance in patients with obstructive sleep apnoea. Thorax 1997;52:648–53.

69. Hack M, Davies RJ, Mullins R, et al. Randomised prospective parallel trial of therapeutic versus subtherapeutic nasal continuous positive airway pressure on simulated steering performance in patients with obstructive sleep apnoea. Thorax 2000;55(3):224–31.

70. Juniper M, Hack MA, George CF, et al. Steering simulation performance in patients with obstructive sleep apnoea and matched control subjects. Eur Respir J 2000;15(3):590–5.

71. Turkington PM, Sircar M, Allgar V, et al. Relationship between obstructive sleep apnoea, driving simulator performance, and risk of road traffic accidents. Thorax 2001;56(10):800–5.

72. Mazza S, Pepin JL, Naegele B, et al. Most obstructive sleep apnoea patients exhibit vigilance and attention deficits on an extended battery of tests. Eur Respir J 2005;25(1):75–80.

73. Philip P, Sagaspe P, Taillard J, et al. Fatigue, sleepiness, and performance in simulated versus real driving conditions. Sleep 2005;28(12):1511–6.

74. Hoekema A, Stegenga B, Bakker M, et al. Simulated driving in obstructive sleep apnoea-hypopnoea; effects of oral appliances and continuous positive airway pressure. Sleep Breath 2007;11(3):129–38.

75. Pizza F, Contardi S, Ferlisi M, et al. Daytime driving simulation performance and sleepiness in obstructive sleep apnoea patients. Accid Anal Prev 2008; 40(2):602–9.

76. Risser MR, Ware JC, Freeman FG. Driving simulation with EEG monitoring in normal and obstructive sleep apnea patients. Sleep 2000;23(3):393–8.

77. Banks S, Catcheside P, Lack LC, et al. The Maintenance of Wakefulness Test and driving simulator performance. Sleep 2005;28(11):1381–5.

78. Desai AV, Marks GB, Jankelson D, et al. Do sleep deprivation and time of day interact with mild obstructive sleep apnea to worsen performance and neurobehavioral function? J Clin Sleep Med 2006;2(1):63–70.

79. Boyle LN, Tippin J, Paul A, et al. Driver performance in the moments surrounding a microsleep. Transp Res Part F Traffic Psychol Behav 2008; 11(2):126–36.

80. Tassi P, Greneche J, Pebayle T, et al. Are OSAS patients impaired in their driving ability on a circuit with medium traffic density? Accid Anal Prev 2008;40(4):1365–70.

81. Pizza F, Contardi S, Mondini S, et al. Daytime sleepiness and driving performance in patients with obstructive sleep apnea: comparison of the MSLT, the MWT, and a simulated driving task. Sleep 2009;32(3):382–91.

82. Vakulin A, Baulk SD, Catcheside PG, et al. Effects of alcohol and sleep restriction on simulated driving performance in untreated patients with obstructive sleep apnea. Ann Intern Med 2009; 151(7):447–55.

83. Filtness AJ, Reyner LA, Horne JA. Moderate sleep restriction in treated older male OSA participants: greater impairment during monotonous driving compared with controls. Sleep Med 2011;12(9): 838–43.

84. Pizza F, Contardi S, Mondini S, et al. Simulated driving performance coupled with driver behaviour can predict the risk of sleepiness-related car accidents. Thorax 2011;66(8):725–6.

85. Vakulin A, Baulk SD, Catcheside PG, et al. Driving simulator performance remains impaired in patients with severe OSA after CPAP treatment. J Clin Sleep Med 2011;7(3):246–53.

86. Ghosh D, Jamson SL, Baxter PD, et al. Continuous measures of driving performance on an advanced office-based driving simulator can be used to predict simulator task failure in patients with obstructive sleep apnoea syndrome. Thorax 2012;67(9):815–21.

87. Ghosh D, Jamson SL, Baxter PD, et al. Factors that affect simulated driving in patients with obstructive sleep apnoea. ERJ Open Res 2015;1(2).

88. May JF, Porter BE, Ware JC. The deterioration of driving performance over time in drivers with untreated sleep apnea. Accid Anal Prev 2016;89: 95–102.

89. Mazza S, Pepin JL, Naegele B, et al. Driving ability in sleep apnoea patients before and after CPAP treatment: evaluation on a road safety platform. Eur Respir J 2006;28(5):1020–8.

90. Filtness AJ, Reyner LA, Horne JA. One night's CPAP withdrawal in otherwise compliant OSA patients: marked driving impairment but good awareness of increased sleepiness. Sleep Breath 2012; 16(3):865–71.

91. Hallvig D, Anund A, Fors C, et al. Sleepy driving on the real road and in the simulator–A comparison. Accid Anal Prev 2013;50:44–50.

92. Demirdogen Cetinoglu E, Gorek Dilektasli A, Demir NA, et al. The relationship between driving simulation performance and obstructive sleep apnoea risk, daytime sleepiness, obesity and road traffic accident history of commercial drivers in Turkey. Sleep Breath 2015;19(3):865–72.

93. Orth M, Duchna HW, Leidag M, et al. Driving simulator and neuropsychological testing in OSAS before and under CPAP therapy. Eur Respir J 2005;26(5):898–903.

94. Contardi S, Pizza F, Sancisi E, et al. Reliability of a driving simulation task for evaluation of sleepiness. Brain Res Bull 2004;63(5):427–31.

95. Hack MA, Choi SJ, Vijayapalan P, et al. Comparison of the effects of sleep deprivation, alcohol and obstructive sleep apnoea (OSA) on simulated steering performance. Respir Med 2001;95(7): 594–601.

96. Gieteling EW, Bakker MS, Hoekema A, et al. Impaired driving simulation in patients with periodic limb movement disorder and patients with obstructive sleep apnea syndrome. Sleep Med 2012;13(5):517–23.

97. Turkington PM, Sircar M, Saralaya D, et al. Time course of changes in driving simulator performance with and without treatment in patients with sleep apnoea hypopnoea syndrome. Thorax 2004;59(1):56–9.

98. Antonopoulos CN, Sergentanis TN, Daskalopoulou SS, et al. Nasal continuous positive airway pressure (nCPAP) treatment for obstructive sleep apnea, road traffic accidents and driving simulator performance: a meta-analysis. Sleep Med Rev 2011;15(5):301–10.

99. Shiomi T, Arita AT, Sasanabe R, et al. Falling asleep while driving and automobile accidents among patients with obstructive sleep apnea-hypopnea syndrome. Psychiatry Clin Neurosci 2002;56(3):333–4.

100. Tregear S, Reston J, Schoelles K, et al. Obstructive sleep apnea and risk of motor vehicle crash: systematic review and meta-analysis. J Clin Sleep Med 2009;5(6):573–81.

Screening for Sleepiness and Sleep Disorders in Commercial Drivers

Indira Gurubhagavatula, MD, MPH[a,b,*], Shannon S. Sullivan, MD[c]

KEYWORDS

- Screening • Obstructive sleep apnea • Sleep disorders • Commercial drivers
- Occupational sleep medicine

KEY POINTS

- Screening for obstructive sleep apnea in commercial drivers is imperative because it is common, identifiable in the latent stage, associated with drowsiness-related crashes, and treatable.
- Screening should use objective, not subjective measures, because of the potential for misreporting or underreporting of symptoms in occupational settings.
- Guidelines are available for the screening, diagnosis, and management of sleep apnea, which emphasize keeping the driver on the road whenever possible.
- The costs of diagnostic testing have decreased in recent years, with the advent of portable monitoring devices that can be used in the berth.
- Long-term treatment of sleep apnea with continuous positive airway pressure therapy has been shown to reduce crashes, provided the driver adheres to the therapy.

INTRODUCTION

Sleepiness and sleep disorders are common in commercial drivers. Estimates indicate that 2.4 to 3.9 million of the approximately 14 million US commercial drivers have obstructive sleep apnea (OSA).[1] Excessive daytime sleepiness (EDS) affects 10% to 25% of adults,[2] and OSA is the most common medical cause of EDS.[3] Untreated OSA has been associated with a host of safety, performance, and health consequences, including increased crash risk.[4] Although no federal requirement mandates screening or specifies the criteria to be used to screen for OSA in commercial

drivers, we review the multiple available paradigms to address these steps, which were developed by expert panels. Such endeavors are paramount, because the available evidence suggests that finding and treating OSA in commercial drivers decreases crash risk[5] and provides numerous health benefits.

DEFINITION OF SCREENING

Screening may refer to 1 of 2 scenarios. First is population-wide assessment to identify an occult disorder, before the manifestation of overt symptoms and adverse consequences. An example is the use of Papanicolaou smears to screen for the

Disclosure Statement: I. Gurubhagavatula: Recipient of a research grant from BluTech, Inc, to study the role of blue-blocking eyewear on melatonin secretion in healthy adults. Recipient of a research grant from the American Academy of Sleep Medicine Foundation to study sleep apnea in law enforcement officers. S.S. Sullivan has nothing to disclose.
[a] Division of Sleep Medicine, Perelman School of Medicine, University of Pennsylvania, 3624 Market Street, Suite 205, Philadelphia, PA 19104, USA; [b] Sleep Section, Crescenz VA Medical Center, Philadelphia, PA, USA; [c] SleepEval Research Institute, 3430 West Bayshore Road, Palo Alto, CA 94303, USA
* Corresponding author. Division of Sleep Medicine, Perelman School of Medicine, University of Pennsylvania, 3624 Market Street, Suite 205, Philadelphia, PA 19104, USA
E-mail address: gurubhag@pennmedicine.upenn.edu

presence of cervical cancer. A second form of screening involves risk stratification, wherein a simple, inexpensive, or more accessible testing strategy is used to identify individuals at greatest risk for the disorder, who may then be offered confirmatory testing using a gold standard. For example, the enzyme-linked immunosorbent assay is using to screen for HIV, and a positive test is confirmed by Western blot.

A screening test may predict the presence or absence of disease correctly or incorrectly. Therefore, screening may result not only in true positive and true negative predictions, but also false-positive predictions, in which the screening test predicts disease that is not present on gold standard testing, and false-negative predictions, in which the screening test misses the diagnosis altogether. The focus of screening efforts may vary based on the goals of the program. A general wellness program may aim to screen for all potential cases of OSA, so that treatment can offset potential general health consequences. A program mandated by government or an employer, however, may focus efforts on finding only those individuals with OSA who are at risk of having a crash. Although high accuracy is desirable, when treatment is benign and of low risk to the patient, the primary focus of screening for a disorder with serious consequences such as drowsiness-related crashes, is to minimize the risk of false-negative predictions, that is, missed cases.

CHARACTERISTICS THAT DELINEATE AN APPROPRIATE TARGET FOR SCREENING

When choosing to target a disorder for screening, several characteristics are considered ideal: high prevalence, identifiable in the latent stage, a long latent stage, adverse consequences if left unidentified, and the availability of effective treatment.[6] First, the disorder should be common. When population-wide screening is performed for a rare condition, the likelihood that a positive result is a false-positive one increases. The condition should also be identifiable in a latent stage, before the occurrence of consequences, and that latent stage should be long enough to allow time for screening interventions. Once found, the condition should be treatable. Therefore, community-acquired pneumonia would not be a suitable candidate for screening, because of the relatively short latency period. A high-grade malignancy may not be a good target candidate for screening, if it progresses rapidly and if an effective treatment does not exist. Our discussion of screening will focus on OSA, the sleep disorder that has been best-studied in commercial drivers.

OBSTRUCTIVE SLEEP APNEA IS AN IDEAL TARGET FOR SCREENING IN COMMERCIAL DRIVERS

OSA meets the 4 characteristics of a disorder that is suitable for screening. It is highly prevalent, identifiable in the latent stage, has a long period before the development of adverse consequences, and is treatable using first-line positive airway pressure (PAP) therapy.

Obstructive Sleep Apnea Is Common

Several studies have estimated the prevalence of OSA in commercial drivers to range between 28% to 80%.[7–11] The first was performed at Stanford,[10] and found that 80% of drivers employed by a single company had evidence of OSA based on overnight oximetry, which showed intermittent desaturation. In 2 large, community-based cohorts of commercial drivers, 28% of American drivers[9] and 60% of Australian drivers[8] had OSA. Another study included drivers in a large, private trucking company in the United States, and estimated that 21% of drivers had OSA.[7]

Obstructive Sleep Apnea Is Associated with Crashes

An increased risk of crashes related to OSA could be due to overt EDS, inattention, distractibility, impaired judgment, increased risk taking, or slowed reaction time. Pooled data from 10 studies[4] estimated that the odds that a driver with OSA would have a crash was 2.4 times greater than a driver without OSA. In this meta-analysis, 95% of drivers with untreated OSA had an increased crash risk, ranging from 21% to 489% higher than those without OSA. Similarly, data from driving simulators shows that performance impairment in OSA is comparable with impairment from alcohol consumption or sleep deprivation.[12]

EDS itself is a contributing factor in approximately 5% to 7% of all MVAs overall, and in approximately 17% of fatal accidents.[13] In a pan-European analysis of more than 12,000 individuals from 19 countries, a high risk of OSA increased the odds of falling asleep at the wheel by 3.48 times.[14] Extrapolating this risk of EDS from passenger car drivers to commercial drivers has remained challenging, in part because commercial drivers tend to underreport sleepiness in clinical settings.[11,15–18] In 1 research environment, however, involving 714 Portuguese truck drivers, 20%

admitted to EDS and 29% were at high risk for having OSA. In this cohort, 42.5% of near-miss accidents and 16.3% of all accidents were self-attributed to sleepiness. Defined as an Epworth Sleepiness Scale score of 11 or greater, sleepiness was a risk factor for both near-miss accidents (odds ratio, 3.84; $P<.01$) and accidents (odds ratio, 2.25; $P<.01$). A high Mallampati score, an established risk factor for OSA, increased the odds of near-miss accidents (odds ratio, 1.89).[19]

Obstructive Sleep Apnea Can Contribute to Accidents in the Workplace, Lost Time from Work, Lower Productivity, and High Employee Turnover

OSA may lead to an increased risk of injury,[20] decreased productivity,[21] and, based on a recent comprehensive meta-analysis, it may double the odds of workplace accidents.[22] Higher rates of employee turnover, a source of high costs for trucking companies, has also been attributed to OSA.[23] These outcomes result in negative economic consequences,[24–26] and 1 economic analysis showed that screening for the disorder proves to be more cost effective than not screening.[26]

Obstructive Sleep Apnea Can Lead to Adverse Health Consequences

Among general populations, OSA is associated with increased all-cause mortality.[27,28] A meta-analysis of more than 25,000 individuals in 12 studies has demonstrated relative risks of 1.79 for cardiovascular disease, 2.15 for fatal and nonfatal stroke, and 1.92 for death from all causes in persons with OSA.[29] The association between OSA and hypertension is reasonably robust. In the large, prospective, community-based Sleep Health Heart Study, compared with individuals with an apnea–hypopnea index (AHI) of less than 1.5 per hour, the odds of hypertension were 20%, 30%, and 40% higher for individuals in mild (5–15 per hour), moderate (15–30 per hour), and severe (>30 per hour) AHI categories, respectively.[30] OSA is also linked to drug-resistant hypertension.[31] Finally, evidence suggesting that treatment of OSA with PAP reverses daytime hypertension in the first few weeks after starting treatment, strengthens the causal link between OSA and hypertension.[32–34]

OSA has also been associated with diabetes in a prospective evaluation.[35] Individuals with untreated OSA and diabetes have been shown to have poorer control of blood sugar, thus, compounding the risk of further morbidity and mortality. Similarly, cerebrovascular disease is associated with mild to moderate and severe OSA, after accounting for other risk factors such as hypertension, hyperlipidemia, and diabetes.[36]

OSA can also decrease quality of life based on a number of measures, including physical function, vitality, and health perception.[37]

Obstructive Sleep Apnea Is Identifiable

A variety of strategies have been suggested to identify commercial drivers at highest risk for OSA, that is, drivers who should undergo confirmatory diagnostic testing. These include symptoms, obesity-related metrics, upper airway anatomic features, and the presence of OSA-related consequences.

When considering screening strategies in general clinic populations or sleep centers, the first-line approach is to ask the patient about common symptoms of OSA, which include loud, habitual snoring, choking or gasping during sleep, nocturia, morning headaches, and daytime sleepiness, which may be assessed using the subjectively rated Epworth Sleepiness Scale.[38] A variety of screening questionnaires also exist.[39–41] However, in commercial driver populations, subjective reports have been shown to have limited usefulness.[11,15–18] Some have hypothesized that reasons for this underreporting include lack of awareness, or avoidance owing to concerns regarding employability.[18]

POTENTIAL SCREENING STRATEGIES: THE ROLE OF OBJECTIVE CRITERIA

Objectively derived metrics have been more useful in case identification of OSA in commercial drivers, and several such metrics have been suggested as first-line tools in screening protocols in a recent consensus statement.[42] These include body mass index and neck circumference, which are surrogate measures of obesity and central obesity, respectively. Other objective signs include resistant hypertension, retrognathia or micrognathia, large tongue, enlarged tonsils, or crowded airway. Obesity in the setting of type 2 diabetes has been proposed as another clue to identifying high-risk individuals, because this combination has been associated with an 80% prevalence of OSA.[43]

A number of other guidance documents, similarly, advocate for the use of objective criteria and emphasize body mass index in particular. Threshold values, including a body mass index of 30 or greater,[44] 33,[45] 35,[46] and 40[42] kg/m² have been proposed. Although higher thresholds offer greater specificity, they also run the risk of missing cases of OSA, which may still lead to crashes. Lower thresholds, in contrast, have not gained wide acceptance because they would require many more drivers to be tested, which could pose logistical and economic challenges.

DIAGNOSTIC CONFIRMATION: ROLE OF PORTABLE MONITORING

Once a commercial driver has been identified to be at high risk, confirmatory diagnostic testing should be offered. Traditionally, such testing has required the driver to spend 1 or sometimes 2 nights in a sleep laboratory to undergo polysomnography (PSG) to test for the frequency of breathing stops (apneas) or airflow reductions (hypopneas) that result in decreases in oxygen saturation by a pre-defined threshold[47] or an arousal from sleep. This method of confirmation required that drivers sleep in a laboratory, which posed logistical challenges for long-haul drivers, and carried the problem of decreased access and long wait times, during which crash risk persisted. Drivers undergoing preemployment evaluation, or deemed to be at high risk for a crash (discussed elsewhere in this article) and advised to stop driving until treatment may lose wages during this period.

In recent years, home-based sleep apnea testing strategies have emerged,[48,49] which are more accessible, less expensive, can be self-assembled, and can be done directly in the berths of trucks or at home. These tests, however, do not measure sleep, but use test duration and subjectively reported diaries to estimate sleep time. The lack of monitoring for sleep can also result in an underestimation of hypopneas, which sometimes lead to arousal even in the absence of significant oxyhemoglobin desaturation, and thereby contribute to daytime sleepiness and its attendant consequences. Furthermore, the lack of ability to track who the wearer is means that a negative test may require further evaluation in a sleep laboratory; because home-based sleep apnea testing is offered to individuals who are already at high risk, a negative result is more likely to be a false negative and requires additional follow-up testing, either at home or in the laboratory.

THE ROLE OF POSITIVE AIRWAY PRESSURE IN RISK REDUCTION

Use of PAP has been shown to decrease excess crash risk associated with OSA; specifically, PAP treatment of OSA has been demonstrated to lower crash risk to the same level as that seen in individuals without OSA, improve sleepiness, and improve performance on a driving simulator. The latter improvements may be seen very quickly, within a matter of days.[5] In 1 study within a single large trucking company, 1603 commercial truck drivers with OSA confirmed by PSG were compared with 403 drivers without OSA by PSG and 2016 matched control drivers who were deemed unlikely to have OSA. PAP was offered to drivers with PSG-confirmed OSA, and adherence rates based on data downloaded from PAP devices were tracked, with Department of Transportation–reported crashes per 100,000 miles driven. The crash rate among drivers with OSA who were not using PAP was 5-fold higher than that of drivers without OSA. The crash rate among drivers with OSA who used PAP was similar to the crash rate in the control group.[23] In follow-up, of 255 commercial truck drivers with a diagnosis of OSA treated with PAP, 75% had a preventable crash during the full study period (before and after PAP). Among those with crashes, the crash was timed before treatment in 93%, whereas 25% were involved in a crash after PAP treatment (thus, a 73% decrease in total crashes). In this study, 91% of drivers assessed for PAP adherence were using PAP therapy 6 to 7 nights per week. Despite the lack of detail regarding AHI, the report indicated that 44% of drivers with a diagnosis of OSA at the single testing site had severe OSA (AHI range from 34 to 112 events per hour of sleep).[50] These data parallel findings in noncommercial drivers, in whom vehicular crashes and fatalities decrease with treatment of OSA.[23,51,52]

In addition to lowering crash risk, PAP therapy has been linked with average savings in health care expenditures of $550 per driver per month, a decrease in hospital admissions by 25%, and in total health care cost by 50%.[53]

RISK ASSESSMENT DURING POSITIVE AIRWAY PRESSURE TREATMENT

Guidance on thresholds for the use of PAP in commercial drivers has been offered, with the goal of mitigating risk while also keeping the driver on the road whenever possible. Despite its imperfections as a metric for severity of disease, the AHI has been used as an important marker in the identification of commercial drivers requiring treatment. Given the lack of specific Federal Motor Carrier Safety Administration requirements pertaining to this metric, a collection of medical consensus recommendations have been offered that aim to reflect current standards of care.[54] Some of these consensus conferences included a Tri-Society Joint Task Force,[55] a Medical Expert Panel[45] commissioned by the Federal Motor Carrier Safety Administration, and combined Motor Carrier Safety Advisory Committee-Medical Review Board in 2012[46] and 2016. The Tri-Society

Joint Task Force recommended an initial threshold for required treatment of an AHI of greater than 30, and all subsequent groups, as well as the American Academy of Sleep Medicine,[42] have recommended a threshold for required OSA treatment of an AHI or 20 or more events per hour. Data linking crash risk are more consistent in moderate to severe AHI ranges than in the mild AHI range (<15 events per hour).[4] Most of the consensus guidelines suggest using a still lower threshold value of AHI for mandatory treatment in particular situations, including serious comorbidity, severe desaturation or sleepiness, or a history of a crash. These thresholds are derived from in-laboratory PSG rather than home testing. Because home testing may underestimate severity, the use of clinical judgment in addition to AHI threshold is advised.

For drivers with moderate-to-severe apnea, PAP therapy is recommended as primary therapy because of its effectiveness in improving health, safety, and costs. As noted, PAP offers salient benefits in the occupational benefits, as it decrease crash risk in commercial drivers with OSA,[5,23,51] decrease the costs of health care[56] and disability,[56,57] and improves mortality.[58]

NON–POSITIVE AIRWAY PRESSURE THERAPIES FOR OBSTRUCTIVE SLEEP APNEA IN COMMERCIAL DRIVERS: SPECIAL CONSIDERATIONS

Non-PAP therapies or combined therapy options for OSA are available for subgroups of commercial drivers. These treatment options include mandibular advancement devices,[59] upper airway surgery of soft tissues or jaw,[60] hypoglossal nerve stimulation to augment inspiratory airway muscle dilation during sleep,[61] positional therapy and weight loss, including weight loss surgeries.[62] These treatment options are available for those with milder AHI values, or for those who have had difficulty tolerating PAP therapy.

SCREENING FOR RESIDUAL CRASH RISK DURING TREATMENT

Once a commercial driver with OSA receives therapy, ongoing screening for residual crash risk is warranted, with an assessment of suitability to continue driving. In this regard, an evaluation of the efficacy of treatment is helpful, and must address adherence, as well as improvement in apneas and hypopneas and reduction of associated clinical findings to acceptable levels. A combination of physician judgment, symptoms, objective testing, and adherence data are helpful in making

this determination. Consensus recommendations advise that commercial drivers with OSA have at least annual follow-up with a board-certified sleep medicine specialist.[42]

PAP devices have built-in compliance and efficacy monitoring systems; recent PAP models transmit this data wirelessly, which is available remotely, and systems are available to cue providers when inadequate treatment efficacy is observed. Although these technologies are evolving, daily monitoring for usage and/or efficacy is unavailable for non-PAP therapies such as oral appliances and positional treatment devices. When these therapies are used, a sleep study may be performed while the patient uses the intervention, which provides a single night's assessment of efficacy. Current clinical guidelines advocate that OSA-related therapies target a decrease in the apnea-hypopnea frequency to fewer than 5 events per hour of sleep.[42] For those whose post-treatment values are 5 to 20 events per hour, clinical judgment is needed to determine fitness for duty. Most data have relied on in-laboratory assessment of apneas and hypopneas per hour of sleep; the optimal threshold values to use with home-based testing are not specified, and these do not measure sleep duration but rather test time.

Data from both commercial and noncommercial drivers shows that close follow-up of recently diagnosed patients improves long-term adherence to treatment.[63] Second, improved adherence to PAP is associated with greater normalization in subjective and objective measures of sleepiness as well as sleep-related quality of life,[64] and may result in greater employee retention.[23]

Current guidelines recommend that adherence to PAP therapies be defined as use of PAP for 4 hours or more per night for 70% or more of nights, for at least 1 week when initiating therapy, or to reinstitute to full service if the driver has been temporarily disqualified from driving.[42,45,46,54,55] However, longer periods of use of these devices, that is, for the full duration of sleep, is expected to provide greater improvements in sleepiness and daytime functioning.

Approaches in the determination of fitness for duty when OSA has been diagnosed in commercial drivers are shown in **Table 1**.[42] In general, a commercial driver with an OSA diagnosis would not be restricted from driving if (1) the AHI is less than 20 events per hour, and (2) excessive sleepiness during the major wake period is not reported; or (3) there is documented efficacy of treatment, including both adherence and effectiveness. In contrast, immediate suspension from duty is recommended if (1) excessive

Table 1
Criteria to assess fitness to drive for safety-sensitive workers who are suspected of having or have OSA

No Restrictions	Conditional Certification	Immediate Suspension

A worker with an OSA diagnosis would NOT receive restrictions if the following conditions are met:
1. The worker has untreated OSA with AHI <20 events per hour, and does not report excess sleepiness during the major wake period, or
2. The worker has OSA (any AHI), and treatment efficacy has been documented:
  a. The worker does not report experiencing excess sleepiness during the major wake period, and
  b. Meets minimal acceptable adherence levels with treatment (average of ≥4 hours of use per day on ≥70% of days)
Workers should be made aware that optimal benefits of PAP therapy occur with ≥7 hours of daily use.
	Neither meets conditions for immediate disqualification, nor for unrestricted driving, and any of the following conditions are met:
	1. The worker has screened positive for possible OSA and is waiting to have a sleep study
	2. The worker has an AHI ≥20 events per hour until adherence with PAP is established
	Conditional restrictions include the following elements:
	1. A worker who screened positive for possible OSA may continue their safety-sensitive work for 60 d pending sleep study and treatment (if diagnosis of OSA is made)
	2. After PAP therapy is initiated for OSA, he or she may return to safety-sensitive work after a minimum of 1 week of demonstrated adherence and treatment efficacy. This conditional period should be limited to 30 days
	  a. Once 30 days have elapsed, if the certifying clinician finds continued adherence and treatment efficacy, this conditional period may be extended by a further 60 days
	  b. At the end of the 60-day extension, if the worker demonstrates adherence and treatment efficacy, certification may be issued with reevaluation at least yearly
	  c. Treatment efficacy should be determined by the treating provider, and includes and assessment of adherence and efficacy of CPAP, which includes assessment for mask leak, residual sleep disordered breathing events on the download, and clinical response, with the caveat that absence of symptoms may be unreliable
		Workers should be disqualified immediately from engaging in safety-sensitive duties if any of the following conditions are met:
		1. The worker reports experiencing excessive sleepiness during the major wake period while engaging in safety-sensitive duties, or
		2. The worker experienced an accident associated with drowsiness, or
		3. The worker fell asleep while performing a safety-sensitive duty, or
		4. The worker is found to be nonadherent with treatment recommendations or follow-up, and has an AHI of ≥20 events per hour, or is deemed to have severe OSA based on clinical manifestations other than AHI (severe desaturation, comorbidities)
		Employers should work with health care professionals to develop policies to manage patients with very severe OSA, in whom even a single night without PAP use are judged to pose significant risk.

(continued on next page)

No Restrictions	Conditional Certification	Immediate Suspension
Table 1 *(continued)*		
	3. The worker who has undergone upper airway surgical treatment should remain out of service until reevaluated after a recovery period of ≥90 days. Reevaluation includes a postoperative sleep study. Further restrictions, if any, would be based on the aforementioned criteria. Workers who undergo bariatric surgery should be reevaluated once weight nadir is reached, to assess for ongoing need for PAP therapy.	

Abbreviation: CPAP, continuous positive airway pressure.

From Gurubhagavatula I, Sullivan S, Meoli A, Patil S, Olson R, Berneking M, et al. Management of Obstructive Sleep Apnea in Commercial Motor Vehicle Operators: Recommendations of the AASM Sleep and Transportation Safety Awareness Task Force. J Clin Sleep Med. 2017;13:745-58; with permission.

sleepiness while performing safety sensitive duties is present; or (2) there is a history of an accident in which drowsiness was implicated; or (3) the worker fell asleep while performing a safety sensitive duty; or (4) there is an AHI of 20 or more events per hour and the driver is noncompliant with treatment recommendations or follow-up; or (5) the driver is deemed to have severe OSA based on clinical manifestations other than AHI (eg, degree of desaturation, comorbidity), until treatment efficacy is established. Conditional certification in 30- to 60-day increments may be offered between screening positive for OSA but before testing; or between diagnosis and the establishment of treatment efficacy, as detailed in **Table 1**. If upper airway surgery is offered in place of PAP, time away from service may be longer because repeat testing to establish efficacy is recommended to occur at least 90 days after the surgical intervention.[42]

SUMMARY

OSA is common among commercial drivers, who tend to be male, middle-aged, and obese, which are key risk factors for the disorder. Left untreated, OSA can lead to serious fall asleep crashes that result in injury, death, and financial loss. OSA is identifiable, and inexpensive strategies now exist to identify high-risk drivers and get them treated. Treatment, in the form PAP, is effective and can reduce crash risk, and requires ongoing support to ensure adherence and efficacy. Most drivers

identified to have OSA can be effectively managed and continue be employed as occupational drivers.

The future continues to evolve quickly in this area, given the rapid pace of technological advances. These include in-vehicle, real-time alertness monitoring methodologies; more comprehensive portable diagnostic testing strategies that minimize data loss and inaccuracy, including sleep time and incorporating chain of custody tracking; smaller and more comfortable PAP therapy devices that increase user acceptance and engagement; telemedicine strategies to increase access and convenience to long-haul drivers and those in remote geographic areas; and autonomous or semiautonomous vehicles, which have alertness management programs to enhance safety.

Ultimately, OSA in commercial drivers is a common, serious disorder that is both identifiable and treatable. Addressing the disorder through proactive screening and treatment aimed at crash risk reduction has the potential to improve the overall health of the driver, while also enhancing public safety for all drivers.

REFERENCES

1. Kales SN, Straubel MG. Obstructive sleep apnea in North American commercial drivers. Ind Health 2014;52:13–24.
2. Ferini-Strambi L, Sforza M, Poletti M, et al. Daytime sleepiness: more than just obstructive sleep apnea (OSA). Med Lav 2017;108:260–6.

3. Kales SN. Preventing Accidents in North American Commercial Drivers with Obstructive Sleep Apnea. Summary of Remarks, Transport Safety Public Symposium of the International Association of Traffic and Safety Sciences. Tokyo, May 20, 2013.

4. Tregear S, Reston J, Schoelles K, et al. Obstructive sleep apnea and risk of motor vehicle crash: systematic review and meta-analysis. J Clin Sleep Med 2009;5:573–81.

5. Tregear S, Reston J, Schoelles K, et al. Continuous positive airway pressure reduces risk of motor vehicle crash among drivers with obstructive sleep apnea: systematic review and meta-analysis. Sleep 2010;33:1373–80.

6. Baumel MJ, Maislin G, Pack AI. Population and occupational screening for obstructive sleep apnea: are we there yet? Am J Respir Crit Care Med 1997;155:9–14.

7. Berger M, Varvarigou V, Rielly A, et al. Employer-mandated sleep apnea screening and diagnosis in commercial drivers. J Occup Environ Med 2012;54:1017–25.

8. Howard ME, Desai AV, Grunstein RR, et al. Sleepiness, sleep-disordered breathing, and accident risk factors in commercial vehicle drivers. Am J Respir Crit Care Med 2004;170:1014–21.

9. Pack A, Dinges D, Maislin G. A study of prevalence of sleep apnea among commercial truck drivers. Washington, DC: Federal Motor Carrier Safety Administration; 2002.

10. Stoohs RA, Bingham LA, Itoi A, et al. Sleep and sleep-disordered breathing in commercial long-haul truck drivers. Chest 1995;107:1275–82.

11. Platt AB, Wick LC, Hurley S, et al. Hits and misses: screening commercial drivers for obstructive sleep apnea using guidelines recommended by a joint task force. J Occup Environ Med 2013;55:1035–40.

12. Tippin J. Driving impairment in patients with obstructive sleep apnea syndrome. Am J Electroneurodiagnostic Technol 2007;47:114–26.

13. Tefft BC. Prevalence of motor vehicle crashes involving drowsy drivers, United States, 1999-2008. Accid Anal Prev 2012;45:180–6.

14. Goncalves M, Amici R, Lucas R, et al. Sleepiness at the wheel across Europe: a survey of 19 countries. J Sleep Res 2015;24:242–53.

15. Dagan Y, Doljansky JT, Green A, et al. Body Mass Index (BMI) as a first-line screening criterion for detection of excessive daytime sleepiness among professional drivers. Traffic Inj Prev 2006;7:44–8.

16. Xie W, Chakrabarty S, Levine R, et al. Factors associated with obstructive sleep apnea among commercial motor vehicle drivers. J Occup Environ Med 2011;53:169–73.

17. Parks P, Durand G, Tsismenakis AJ, et al. Screening for obstructive sleep apnea during commercial driver medical examinations. J Occup Environ Med 2009;51:275–82.

18. Talmage JB, Hudson TB, Hegmann KT, et al. Consensus criteria for screening commercial drivers for obstructive sleep apnea: evidence of efficacy. J Occup Environ Med 2008;50:324–9.

19. Catarino R, Spratley J, Catarino I, et al. Sleepiness and sleep-disordered breathing in truck drivers : risk analysis of road accidents. Sleep Breath 2014;18:59–68.

20. Sanna A. Obstructive sleep apnoea, motor vehicle accidents, and work performance. Chron Respir Dis 2013;10:29–33.

21. Mulgrew AT, Ryan CF, Fleetham JA, et al. The impact of obstructive sleep apnea and daytime sleepiness on work limitation. Sleep Med 2007;9:42–53.

22. Garbarino S, Guglielmi O, Sanna A, et al. Risk of occupational accidents in workers with obstructive sleep apnea: systematic review and meta-analysis. Sleep 2016;39:1211–8.

23. Burks SV, Anderson JE, Bombyk M, et al. Nonadherence with employer-mandated sleep apnea treatment and increased risk of serious truck crashes. Sleep 2016;39:967–75.

24. AlGhanim N, Comondore VR, Fleetham J, et al. The economic impact of obstructive sleep apnea. Lung 2008;186:7–12.

25. Frost, Sullivan. Hidden health crisis costing America billions. Underdiagnosing and undertreating obstructive sleep apnea draining healthcare system. Darien, IL: American Academy of Sleep Medicine; 2016. Available at: http://www.aasmnet.org/sleep-apnea-economic-impact.aspx. Accessed September 9, 2019.

26. Gurubhagavatula I, Nkwuo JE, Maislin G, et al. Estimated cost of crashes in commercial drivers supports screening and treatment of obstructive sleep apnea. Accid Anal Prev 2008;40:104–15.

27. Marshall NS, Wong KK, Cullen SR, et al. Sleep apnea and 20-year follow-up for all-cause mortality, stroke, and cancer incidence and mortality in the Busselton Health Study cohort. J Clin Sleep Med 2014;10:355–62.

28. Young T, Finn L, Peppard PE, et al. Sleep disordered breathing and mortality: eighteen-year follow-up of the Wisconsin sleep cohort. Sleep 2008;31:1071–8.

29. Wang X, Ouyang Y, Wang Z, et al. Obstructive sleep apnea and risk of cardiovascular disease and all-cause mortality: a meta-analysis of prospective cohort studies. Int J Cardiol 2013;169:207–14.

30. Nieto FJ, Young TB, Lind BK, et al. Association of sleep-disordered breathing, sleep apnea, and hypertension in a large community-based study. Sleep Heart Health Study. JAMA 2000;283:1829–36.

31. Logan AG, Perlikowski SM, Mente A, et al. High prevalence of unrecognized sleep apnoea in drug-resistant hypertension. J Hypertens 2001;19:2271–7.

32. Young T, Peppard PE, Gottlieb DJ. Epidemiology of obstructive sleep apnea: a population health perspective. Am J Respir Crit Care Med 2002;165:1217–39.

33. Martinez-Garcia MA, Capote F, Campos-Rodriguez F, et al. Effect of CPAP on blood pressure in patients with obstructive sleep apnea and resistant hypertension: the HIPARCO randomized clinical trial. JAMA 2013;310:2407–15.

34. Duran-Cantolla J, Aizpuru F, Montserrat JM, et al. Continuous positive airway pressure as treatment for systemic hypertension in people with obstructive sleep apnoea: randomised controlled trial. BMJ 2010;341:c5991.

35. Botros N, Concato J, Mohsenin V, et al. Obstructive sleep apnea as a risk factor for type 2 diabetes. Am J Med 2009;122:1122–7.

36. Arzt M, Young T, Finn L, et al. Association of sleep-disordered breathing and the occurrence of stroke. Am J Respir Crit Care Med 2005;172:1447–51.

37. Yang EH, Hla KM, McHorney CA, et al. Sleep apnea and quality of life. Sleep 2000;23:535–41.

38. Johns MW. A new method for measuring daytime sleepiness: the Epworth sleepiness scale. Sleep 1991;14:540–5.

39. Maislin G, Pack AI, Kribbs NB, et al. A survey screen for prediction of apnea. Sleep 1995;18:158–66.

40. Chung F, Yegneswaran B, Liao P, et al. STOP questionnaire: a tool to screen patients for obstructive sleep apnea. Anesthesiology 2008;108:812–21.

41. Netzer NC, Stoohs RA, Netzer CM, et al. Using the Berlin Questionnaire to identify patients at risk for the sleep apnea syndrome. Ann Intern Med 1999;131:485–91.

42. Gurubhagavatula I, Sullivan S, Meoli A, et al. Management of obstructive sleep apnea in commercial motor vehicle operators: recommendations of the AASM sleep and transportation safety awareness task force. J Clin Sleep Med 2017;13:745–58.

43. Foster GD, Sanders MH, Millman R, et al. Obstructive sleep apnea among obese patients with type 2 diabetes. Diabetes Care 2009;32:1017–9.

44. Medical review board meeting summary. Washington, DC: Federal Motor Carrier Safety Administration; 2008. Available at: https://www.fmcsa.dot.gov/sites/fmcsa.dot.gov/files/docs/Fin_Meet_Min_Jan28_2008MRB_Meet_Revised11-24-09.pdf. Accessed January 30, 2019.

45. Ancoli-Israel S, Czeisler CA, George CFP, et al. Expert panel recommendations: obstructive sleep apnea and commercial motor vehicle driver safety. Washington, DC: Federal Motor Carrier Safety Administration; 2008. Available at: https://cms.fmcsa.dot.gov/regulations/medical/expert-panel-recommendations-obstructive-sleep-apnea-and-commercial-motor. Accessed January 30, 2019.

46. Parker DR, Hoffman BH. Motor carrier safety advisory committee and medical review board task 11-05 report. Washington DC: Federal Motor Carrier Safety Administration; 2012. Available at: https://www.fmcsa.dot.gov/february-6-2012-mcsac-and-mrb-task-11-05-final-report-obstructive-sleep-apnea-osa. Accessed September 9, 2019.

47. Kapur VK, Auckley DH, Chowdhuri S, et al. Clinical practice guideline for diagnostic testing for adult obstructive sleep apnea: an American Academy of Sleep Medicine clinical practice guideline. J Clin Sleep Med 2017;13:479–504.

48. Zhang C, Berger M, Malhotra A, et al. Portable diagnostic devices for identifying obstructive sleep apnea among commercial motor vehicle drivers: considerations and unanswered questions. Sleep 2012;35:1481–9.

49. Gurubhagavatula I. Does the rubber meet the road? Addressing sleep apnea in commercial truck drivers. Sleep 2012;35:1443–4.

50. 2015 pocket guide to large truck and bus statistics. Federal Motor Carrier Safety Administration 2015. Available at: https://www.fmcsa.dot.gov/sites/fmcsa.dot.gov/files/docs/2015%20Pocket%20Guide%20-%20March%2030%202015%20%28For%20Web%20Publishing%29-508c_0.pdf. Accessed January 30, 2019.

51. Sassani A, Findley LJ, Kryger M, et al. Reducing motor-vehicle collisions, costs, and fatalities by treating obstructive sleep apnea syndrome. Sleep 2004;27:453–8.

52. Karimi M, Hedner J, Habel H, et al. Sleep apnea-related risk of motor vehicle accidents is reduced by continuous positive airway pressure: Swedish Traffic Accident Registry data. Sleep 2015;38:341–9.

53. Berger MB, Sullivan W, Owen R, et al. A corporate driven sleep apnea detection and treatment program: results and challenges. Chest 2006;130:157S.

54. Colvin LJ, Collop NA. Commercial motor vehicle driver obstructive sleep apnea screening and treatment in the United States: an update and recommendation overview. J Clin Sleep Med 2016;12:113–25.

55. Hartenbaum N, Collop N, Rosen IM, et al. Sleep apnea and commercial motor vehicle operators: statement from the joint task force of the American College of Chest Physicians, American College of Occupational and Environmental Medicine, and the National Sleep Foundation. J Occup Environ Med 2006;48:S4–37.

56. Potts KJ, Butterfield DT, Sims P, et al. Cost savings associated with an education campaign on the diagnosis and management of sleep-disordered breathing: a retrospective, claims-based US study. Popul Health Manag 2013;16:7–13.

57. Hoffman B, Wingenbach DD, Kagey AN, et al. The long-term health plan and disability cost benefit of obstructive sleep apnea treatment in a commercial motor vehicle driver population. J Occup Environ Med 2010;52:473–7.

58. Barbe F, Duran-Cantolla J, Sanchez-de-la-Torre M, et al. Effect of continuous positive airway pressure on the incidence of hypertension and cardiovascular events in nonsleepy patients with obstructive sleep apnea: a randomized controlled trial. JAMA 2012;307:2161–8.

59. Ramar K, Dort LC, Katz SG, et al. Clinical practice guideline for the treatment of obstructive sleep apnea and snoring with oral appliance therapy: an update for 2015. J Clin Sleep Med 2015;11:773–827.

60. Aurora RN, Casey KR, Kristo D, et al. Practice parameters for the surgical modifications of the upper airway for obstructive sleep apnea in adults. Sleep 2010;33:1408–13.

61. Strollo PJ Jr, Soose RJ, Maurer JT, et al. Upper-airway stimulation for obstructive sleep apnea. N Engl J Med 2014;370:139–49.

62. Hudgel DW, Patel SR, Ahasic AM, et al. The role of weight management in the treatment of adult obstructive sleep apnea. An Official American Thoracic Society clinical practice guideline. Am J Respir Crit Care Med 2018;198:e70–87.

63. Bouloukaki I, Giannadaki K, Mermigkis C, et al. Intensive versus standard follow-up to improve continuous positive airway pressure compliance. Eur Respir J 2014;44:1262–74.

64. Antic NA, Catcheside P, Buchan C, et al. The effect of CPAP in normalizing daytime sleepiness, quality of life, and neurocognitive function in patients with moderate to severe OSA. Sleep 2011; 34:111–9.

Technology to Detect Driver Sleepiness

Thomas Penzel, Dr rer physiol, Dipl Phys[a],*, Ingo Fietze, Dr med[a], Christoph Schöbel, Dr med[b], Christian Veauthier, Dr med[a]

KEYWORDS

- Sleepiness detection • Drowsiness detection • Sensors • Signal analysis

KEY POINTS

- Sleepiness, drowsiness, tiredness, and fatigue need to be defined and distinguished.
- Assessment of sleepiness can be done with electroencephalograms, electrooculograms, and electromyograms in validated tests, such as the multiple sleep latency test and the maintenance of wakefulness test, for which normative values and thresholds are available.
- Correlates for sleepiness, such as reaction time tests, can be used but are less reliable.
- Questionnaires are self-administered and popular measures for perceived sleepiness. They do not correlate well with electroencephalogram-based sleepiness quantification.
- Monitoring of sleepiness at the wheel is possible using technology derived from sleepiness testing.

INTRODUCTION

An assessment of sleepiness first requires a definition of terms, with a focus on vigilance, fatigue, tiredness, sleepiness, and falling asleep. The field of sleep medicine is interested in detecting the transition from wakefulness to sleep by using established equipment for quantifying this process. Electrophysiologic signals are corded on the head, such as with electroencephalograms (EEGs), electrooculograms (EOGs), and electromyograms (EMGs), just as is done during sleep with polysomnography. Because much of the transition from wakefulness to sleep is related to behavior, it is practical and feasible to assess indirect measures of behavior and other correlates of falling asleep as well.[1]

Assessment of sleepiness is of high interest, because drowsiness when driving is causing many accidents. Moreover, the accidents caused often are fatal, because the driver is usually unable to take last-minute actions to prevent the worst outcome. As a consequence, legislation has been installed in Europe to check for sleepiness in patients with the most prevalent sleep disorder, which is sleep apnea.[2] This legislation allows patients with sleep apnea to drive, if treatment is effective to remove sleepiness. An assessment of sleepiness in patients with sleep apnea, and in anybody else, is an important part of sleep medicine testing.

Several overviews on this topic had been published previously as parts of textbooks in the field of sleep medicine.[3–9] A couple of publications focus specifically on drowsiness while driving, present technology to capture falling asleep, and discuss countermeasures.[10] A summary and overview is presented in the white papers.[10]

TERMS AND DEFINITIONS FOR SLEEPINESS

The interest in detecting driver sleepiness is in observing and possibly predicting the transition from wakefulness to sleep. This had been termed,

Disclosure Statement: T. Penzel received research grants by Cidelec, Itamar, Löwenstein Medical, Philips/Respironics, and Resmed. I. Fietze, C. Schöbel, and C. Veauthier have nothing to declare.
[a] Sleep Medicine Center, Charité – Universitätsmedizin Berlin, Charitéplatz 1, Berlin 10117, Germany;
[b] Universitätsmedizin Essen, Ruhrlandklinik - Westdeutsches Lungenzentrum, am Universitätsklinikum Essen gGmbH, Tüschener Weg 40, D-45239 Essen, Germany
* Corresponding author.
E-mail address: thomas.penzel@charite.de

Sleep Med Clin 14 (2019) 463–468
https://doi.org/10.1016/j.jsmc.2019.08.004
1556-407X/19/

vigilance monitoring. A person may report fatigue and tiredness but may not be sleepy and may not tend to fall asleep. In sleep medicine, referring to sleepiness means that a person falls asleep. A person with increased sleepiness falls asleep faster. A shorter sleep-onset latency is observed. This falling asleep quickly may happen even against the intention of the particular person. A driver in a car during night fights against falling asleep and the accompanying person my allow him/herself to fall asleep. When a person is relaxing while watching TV or listening to music, there may be an intention to fall asleep, because this has no negative consequences. A person worrying and stressed by work, however, may want to fall asleep in a relaxing environment and, although very tired, may not be able to do so. This means that boundary conditions and motivation are important modifies to falling asleep. It is not just being tired or being bored when a person is falling asleep. As such, it is not easy to design reliable prediction models for falling asleep at tasks requiring sustained attention, such as driving a car.

In a sleep medicine center, the sleepiness of a subject is quantified. This means that vwith the recording of sleep medicine technology, the sleep-onset latency is quantified, either until a person reaches sleep stage N1 or sleep stage N2. During the sleep laboratory investigation, several factors may influence the sleep latency. These are light, noise, meals and drinks, and stimulating substances, such as coffee or drugs. Accordingly, these conditions need to be documented, and disturbing factors need to be minimized. Medication with consequences for sleepiness may need to be changed prior to testing.

In addition, the subjective sleepiness has to be documented by standardized questionnaires. Standardized questionnaires are discussed later. Sleepiness can be quantified by indirect assessment of performance and reaction time. A sleep laboratory can assess sleepiness in addition to these options with a sleep EEG recording.

QUANTIFY SLEEPINESS WITH SLEEP ELECTROENCEPHALOGRAM RECORDING

The most established method of quantifying sleepiness is the performance of a multiple sleep latency test (MSLT).[11,12] In order to apply an MSLT, a subject is investigated in a sleep center. First a regular sleep recording overnight is done, in order to know the basis on which on the sleepiness is evaluated. Then, the following day, the subject has to undertake a test with the instruction to fall asleep in a bed in the sleep laboratory, with

quiet, dark, and convenient temperature conditions, allowing to fall asleep easily. Two hours after wake-up time, the subject is asked for the first time to perform a sleep latency test. Each single sleep latency test lasts 20 minutes. This partial test is repeated every 2 hours. In total, 4 to 5 test runs with an evaluation of sleep-onset latency are performed. This is where the name, MSLT, comes from. Each test is performed with EEG, EMG, and EOG leads attached, just as during a regular sleep EEG test during the night. Usually, the leads that were used during the night before remain on the head of the patient. Electrode gel is refilled in order to ensure good signal quality during the test recordings. If the subject falls asleep during the test, then the subject is awakened and the test is over. This is done to prevent that subject using the test to sleep and recover. In-between the tests, the subject is not allowed to sleep and is instructed to have regular relaxing activities, such as reading and walking. Healthy subjects who had a restful sleep do not fall asleep or may have a nap after dinner. Sleepy patients do fall asleep several times and maybe within 5 minutes. Finally, sleep latencies from all 4 or 5 tests are averaged. Normal values derived from large groups for sleep latency are available and, therefore, this test is used often.[13] Healthy subjects show a mean sleep latency of 10 minutes to 12 minutes. A subject with a mean sleep latency lower than 5 minutes has highly pathologic daytime sleepiness. A person with a mean sleep latency longer than 15 minutes has no daytime sleepiness. In addition, the sleep onset is evaluated in terms of observing rapid-eye movement (REM) sleep. If a person shows immediate REM sleep, this is called sleep-onset REM. If a person has 2 or more sleep-onset REM episodes, this is a good indication for suffering from narcolepsy. Further diagnostic steps toward narcolepsy should be taken. The MSLT is not useful in patients suffering from insomnia and in patients with circadian sleep-wake rhythm disorders and should not be applied in them.

It could be argued that the instruction "fall asleep" for the MSLT does not reflect the scenario of assessing daytime sleepiness, because the intention of a subject (a driver) is to stay awake and not fall asleep. According to this logic, the maintenance of wakefulness test (MWT) had been designed in close similarity to the MSLT. For the MWT, the instruction is indeed "stay awake." The setting, however, is similar. The test is performed 4 to 5 times, the first time 2 hours after wake-up time, and it should be performed after a reference night in a sleep laboratory with polysomnography. The main difference is the duration of each test run: 40 minutes are given to allow the subject to fall asleep, even when the intention is to stay awake. The environment is similar, again a quiet, dimmed (not totally dark), convenient room and again EEG, EOG, EMG signal recording.[11] An additional minor difference is that the patient is sitting in a chair, not lying in a bed. Large studies, deriving reference values, have determined a threshold of 8 minutes for sleep onset. A subject has an increased daytime sleepiness, if mean sleep-onset latency is 8 minutes or less. The main difference between the tests is that the MWT tests in how far a subject can resist the sleep drive, which builds up during daytime, whereas the MSLT just lets the sleep drive govern and tests whether sleep drive leads to falling asleep. A driver might successfully fight against the sleep drive while the person may fall asleep during MSLT with its different instruction. Both tests do not correlate well with self-reported sleepiness.[14]

Another test to quantify sleepiness with an EEG signal is the Karolinska drowsiness test (KDT). In this test, the person sits in a relaxation chair and looks at a spot or circle on the wall for a given period. This should be a relaxing and boring task. The aim is to check the appearance of alpha waves in the EEG signal and compare them against higher-frequency waves. There are no normative values available, however, for this test. As a result, the test usually is applied to check intraindividual changes of vigilance and sleepiness in a specific test series.

There are various attempts to stage the EEG signal for the transition from wake to sleep.[15,16] Transitions do not fall in a 30-second sleep staging pattern but require adaptive segmentation.[17,18] This had been used to study sleepy patients with obstructive sleep apnea during a sustained 90-minute reaction time test.[19] The test was chosen to be so long that patients used to performing tasks when being sleepy and used to fighting against sleepiness still might become more sleepy and may fall asleep during a boring task.[20,21] For this kind of evaluation, a more detailed classification for the EEG with vigilance stages between bright awake and falling asleep had been defined.[19] This classification is based mainly on the disappearance of beta waves, appearance and disappearance of alpha waves, and the first appearance of theta waves. These stages do not follow a 30-second epoch duration, but EEG patterns determine the beginning and an end of a segment with a certain vigilance stage. A visual staging of this kind of analysis takes a lot of training and a lot of time to do. Therefore, this kind of vigilance staging had been performed only in some research studies and not any further in clinical routine studies.[19]

The recording of EEG while driving had been used to quantify sleepiness at the wheel. This method uses the vigilance staging either based on computer-based pattern recognition[15] or on alpha, beta, and theta wave evaluation with real-time signal processing. New dry EEG electrodes have fueled the development of small devices based on EEG analysis. The required use of head-mounted equipment, however, limits the application of devices in practice to research studies.

QUANTIFY SLEEPINESS WITHOUT SLEEP ELECTROENCEPHALOGRAM RECORDING

Because the recording and evaluation of an EEG requires considerable effort in terms of recording equipment and in terms of specially trained personnel, several tests were developed, which focus on correlates for sleepiness. Most prominent and popular correlates are different variants of reaction time tests. The most well known and most widespread used reaction time test is the psychomotor vigilance test.[22] This test consists of a handheld device with a small light to be completed over a 10-minute test period. If the light lids, a button must be pressed. The reaction time and the number of failures are recorded. The 10 minutes allow checking for a change over time in reaction time and in performance, so an increase in reaction time can be observed in case of severe sleepiness.

A variant of this test is the Oxford sleep resistance test and the multiple unexpected reaction time test.[23,24] Both tests measure the reaction time in response to several visual and auditory signals. Again, the trace of reaction time over the test period shows a progression in case of severe sleepiness. Furthermore, there also are cognitive performance tests in place. The Wiener test system is able to test concentration performance and multitasking ability to react to different stimuli at the same time. Speed of stimuli accelerates at the different test runs so that the subject tested fails in the end of each test run. Reaction time and failure rates are logged and analyzed. All these tests are possibly impaired by the subject motivation and may be subject to faked drowsiness or attention depending on subject motivation.

Testing of sleepiness while driving with visual or acoustic stimuli in order to check reaction time is implemented in trains to check the vigilance of the driver. The test must be simple so that the driver is not distracted from the driving task. If the vigilance task, for example, regular reaction time checking is simple, however, trained drivers can do this half asleep. This has been shown in studies on train drivers.

Video monitoring of a driver allows to check eye movements and eyelid closure. PERCLOS (percentage of eye closure) is a measure derived from video monitoring of the eye.[25] Perclos determines the percentage the eye is closed by the eyelid and can be calculated in real time with cameras installed in the car driver's cockpit. This technology had been implemented in luxury cars and is able to alert the driver and propose counteractions.

In order to reduce the influence of motivation, other procedures try to record physiologic correlates of sleepiness and attention. One such correlate is sympathetic nervous activity. A testing of this activity during daytime is the investigation of the pupil reflexes in the darkness. This method is called pupillography.[26] This measurement cannot be faked as it is hardly influenced by motivation. As a physiologic correlate for sympathetic activity, however, the test is influenced by substances, such as stimulants, drugs, medication, and psychological factors, such as stress. In sum, it is another correlate for sleepiness and has some correlation with drowsiness when driving. It should not be used as a final test to determine the ability of a person to drive or not to drive.

Based on the idea that sympathetic tone declines with sleepiness and getting more drowsy, some approaches have used heart rate processing to predict sleepiness with some success.[27] To derive heart rate from a driver in a moving car seems challenging because steady movements induce so many signal artifacts that the calculation of heart rate becomes unreliable.

SUBJECTIVE SLEEPINESS ASSESSMENT

Questionnaires are popular and well-established methods to assess sleepiness with less methodological effort and less costs. Self-administered questionnaires and observer-based questionnaires can be used.[28] This article presents self-administered questionnaires. The most widespread questionnaire in use is the Epworth Sleepiness Scale (ESS).[29] This questionnaire asks for sleepiness as occurred during the last 4 weeks. There are 8 questions with different falling asleep scenarios and for each of them a value between zero and three should be scored.[29] All scores are then added up. For sum scores of 10 and larger, sleepiness is increased.[30] If, however, instantaneous sleepiness needs to be assessed, maybe to evaluate sleepiness during a driving task, then appropriate questionnaires are Karolinska Sleepiness Scale (KSS) and Stanford Sleepiness Scale.

Actually, both SSS and KSS scales are a score because of having only one question: How sleepy are you now? Both scales allow just one score, with values between 1 and 9 to score the perceived degree of sleepiness. There extremes are extreme awake and very sleepy, fighting against falling asleep. Depending on the test and the situation, one of the questionnaires or scores are applied.

Unfortunately, the ESS does not correlate well with sleepiness as determined by MSLT or MWT.[31] Therefore, many approaches were taken to either improve the questionnaire or to find combinations of tests. A relatively recent and well evaluated variant is the Sleepiness-Wakefulness Inability and Fatigue Test questionnaire.[32–35] This is a 12-item self-administered questionnaire. Some of the items are the same as the ESS items. The questionnaire assesses general wakefulness inability and fatigue and driver wakefulness inability and fatigue. This questionnaire is superior compared with the ESS in terms of sensitivity and specificity. It is strongly recommended to apply this new self-administered test in the assessment of drivers because the test correlates well with continuous positive airway pressure in patients with sleep apnea. This test has not reached a wider distribution and recognition, however, until now.

Sometimes driving simulators are used to determine drowsiness when driving. Many simple driving simulators are available and they resemble computer games. Some driving simulators are sophisticated and expensive and consist of a car chassis, large video screens, and movie-like driving scenarios to produce a more realistic environment for the subject. Comparisons of these simulators did show, however, that independent of sophistication and costs, the examined person does not really forget about the test situation and, as such, the results are similar between different driving simulators and do not differ much when it is related to their performance. Individual subject motivation to fail or pass the test is a much stronger modifier for the results.

SUMMARY

For the quantitative detection of sleepiness in a driver, a good definition and description of the terms are needed first. Sleepiness, drowsiness, tiredness, and fatigue are terms and conditions used in this context and they need to be defined so that they can be distinguished. A quantitative assessment of sleepiness can be done with EEG, EOG, and EMG in a sleep laboratory setting under test conditions. The tests performed are the MSLT and the MWT. Both tests require a sleep recording the night before, so that baseline conditions are specified. For these 2 tests, normative values and thresholds are available. These 2 tests serve as references for quantitative assessment of daytime sleepiness and drowsiness. Correlates for sleepiness, such as reaction time tests, can be used but are less reliable. The most popular test based on reaction time, is the psychomotor vigilance test, which assesses reaction time over a 10-minute period. Normative values for everybody are not available. Questionnaires are self-administered and popular measures for perceived sleepiness. The most widespread questionnaire in use is the ESS. Self-assessed sleepiness, such as the ESS, however, does not necessarily correlate well with EEG-based sleepiness quantification. Driver drowsiness assessment is an important part of sleep laboratory testing, because EU regulations require an assessment due to risk of accidents in patients with sleep disorders and sleep apnea, in particular.

REFERENCES

1. Akerstedt T, Gillberg M. Subjective and objective sleepiness in the active individual. Int J Neurosci 1990;52:29–37.
2. Bonsignore MR, Randerath W, Riha R, et al. New rules on driver licensing for patients with obstructive sleep apnea: European Union Directive 2014/85/EU. J Sleep Res 2016;25:3–4.
3. Mathis J, de Lacy S, Roth C. Assessment of sleep disorders and diagnostic procedures. Measuring – monitoring sleep and wakefulness. In: Bassetti C, Dogas Z, Peigneux P, editors. Sleep medicine textbook. Regensburg, (Germany): European Sleep Research Society; 2014. p. 125–43.
4. Mayer G, Arzt M, Braumann B, et al. S3-Leitlinie Nicht erholsamer Schlaf/Schlafstörungen – Kapitel „Schlafbezogene Atmungsstörungen". Somnologie (Berl) 2017;20(Suppl 2):S97–180.
5. Penzel T, Hirshkowitz M, Harsh J, et al. Digital analysis and technical specifications. J Clin Sleep Med 2007;3:109–20.
6. Penzel T, Brandenburg U, Fischer J, et al. Empfehlungen zur computergestützten Aufzeichnung und Auswertung von Polygraphien. Somnologie (Berl) 1998;2:42–8.
7. Qaseem A, Dallas P, Owens DK, et al, for the clinical guidelines committee of the American college of physicians. Diagnosis of obstructive sleep apnea in adults: a clinical practice guideline from the American college of physicians. Ann Intern Med 2014; 161:210–20.
8. Rechtschaffen A, Kales A. A manual of standardized terminology, techniques and scoring system for sleep stages of human subjects. Los Angeles (CA): UCLA Brain Information Service/Brain Research Institute; 1968.
9. Hirshkowitz M. Polysomnography Challenges. Sleep Med Clinics 2016;11:403–11.
10. Akerstedt T, Bassetti C, Cirignotta F, et al. Sleepiness at the wheel. White paper. Professional Assoc of Toll Road Comp (ASFA) 2013. Available at: http://www.wcommunication.fr/Travaux-edition/Livres-livrets/asfa-livre-blanc-la-somnolence-au-volant-white-paper-sleepiness-at-the-wheel.html. Accessed March 17, 2019.
11. Arand D, Bonnet M, Hurwitz T, et al. The clinical use of the MSLT and the MWT. Sleep 2005;28:123–44.
12. Berry RB, Brooks R, Gamaldo CE, et al, for the American Academy of Sleep Medicine. The AASM manual for the scoring of sleep and associated events: rules, terminology and technical specifications, version 2.5. Darien (IL): American Academy of Sleep Medicine; 2018.
13. Littner MR, Kushida C, Wise M, et al. Practice parameters for clinical use of the multiple sleep latency test and the maintenance of wakefulness test. Sleep 2005;28:113–21.
14. Sangal RB, Thomas L, Mitler MM. Dsorders of excessive sleepiness: treatment improves ability to stay awake but does not reduce sleepiness. Chest 1992;102:699–703.
15. Hasan J, Hirvonen K, Värri A, et al. Validation of computer analysed polygraphic pattern during drowsiness and sleep onset. Electroencephalogr Clin Neurophysiol 1993;87:117–27.
16. Higgins JS, Michael J, Austin R, et al. Asleep at the wheel – the road to addressing drowsy driving. Sleep 2017. https://doi.org/10.1093/sleep/zsx001.
17. Torsvall L, Akerstedt T. Sleepiness on the job: continuously measured EEG changes in train drivers. Electroencephalogr Clin Neurophysiol 1987;66: 502–11.
18. Weess HG, Sauter C, Geisler P, et al. Vigilanz, Einschlafneigung, Daueraufmerksamkeit, Müdigkeit, Schläfrigkeit – Diagnostische Instrumentarien zur Messung müdigkeits- und schläfrigkeitsbezogener Prozesse und deren Gütekriterien. Somnologie (Berl) 2000;4:20–38.
19. Conradt R, Brandenburg U, Penzel T, et al. Vigilance transitions in reaction time test: a method of describing the state of alertness more objectively. Clin Neurophysiol 1999;110:1499–509.
20. Cassel W, Ploch T, Becker C, et al. Risk of traffic accidents in patients with sleep disordered breathing: reduction with nCPAP. Eur Respir J 1996;9: 519–24.
21. Conradt R, Hochban W, Heitmann J, et al. Sleep fragmentation and daytime vigilance in patients with OSA treated by surgical maxillomandibular advancement compared to CPAP therapy. J Sleep Res 1998;7:217–23.

22. Dinges DF, Powell JW. Microcomputer analysis of performance on a portable, simple visual task during sustained operations. Behav Res Methods Instrum Comput 1985;17:652–5.

23. Alakuijala A, Maasilta P, Bachour A. The Oxford Sleep Resistance Test (OSLER) and the multiple unprepared reaction time test (MURT) detect vigilance modifi cations in sleep apnea patients. J Clin Sleep Med 2014;10:1075–82.

24. American Academy of Sleep Medicine (AASM). International Classification of Sleep Disorders (ICSD). 3rd edition. Rochester, (MN): American Academy of Sleep Medicine; 2014.

25. Abe T, Nonomura T, Komada Y, et al. Detecting deteriorated vigilance using percentage of eyelid closure time during behavioral maintenance of wakefulness tests. Int J Psychophysiol 2011;82:269–74.

26. Wilhelm B, Giedke H, Lüdtke H, et al. Daytime variations in central nervous system activation measured by a pupillographic sleepiness test. J Sleep Res 2001;10:1–7.

27. Chua EC, Tan WQ, Yeo SC, et al. Heart rate variability can be used to estimate sleepiness-related decrements in psychomotor vigilance during total sleep deprivation. Sleep 2012;35:325–34.

28. Hirshkowitz M, Sharafkhaneh A. Evaluating sleepiness. In: Kryger M, Roth T, Dement WC, editors. Principles and practice of sleep medicine. 6th edition. Philadelphia: Elsevier; 2017. p. 1651–8.

29. Johns MW. A new method for measuring daytime sleepiness: the Epworth Sleepiness Scale. Sleep 1991;14:540–5.

30. Johns MW. Reliability and factor analysis of the Epworth sleepiness scale. Sleep 1992;15:376–81.

31. Chervin RD. The multiple sleep latency test and Epworth Sleepiness scale in the assessment of daytime sleepiness. J Sleep Res 2000;9:399–401.

32. Sangal RB. Evaluating sleepiness-related daytime function by querying wakefulness inability and fatigue: Sleepiness-Wakefulness Inability and Fatigue Test (SWIFT). J Clin Sleep Med 2012;8:701–11.

33. Shokoueinejad M, Fernandez C, Carroll E, et al. Sleep apnea: a review of diagnostic sensors, algorithms, and therapies. Physiol Meas 2017;38:R204–52.

34. Silber MH, Ancoli-Israel S, Bonnet MH, et al. The visual scoring of sleep in adults. J Clin Sleep Med 2007;3:121–31.

35. Smith MT, McCrae CS, Cheung J, et al. Use of actigraphy for the evaluation of sleep disorders and circadian rhythm sleep-wake disorders: an American Academy of Sleep Medicine clinical practice guideline. J Clin Sleep Med 2018;14:1231–7.

Sleepiness and Driving
Benefits of Treatment

Catherine A. McCall, MD[a,b],*, Nathaniel F. Watson, MD, MSc[c,1]

KEYWORDS

- Drowsy driving • Sleep deprivation • Sleep disorders • Sleep disorder treatment
- Drowsy driving countermeasures

KEY POINTS

- Drowsy driving is an enormous public health issue resulting in significant morbidity, mortality, and economic cost to individuals and society.
- Causes of drowsy driving include acute or chronic sleep deprivation, driving at inappropriate times in the circadian cycle, untreated sleep disorders, other medical or psychiatric disorders, and medication/substance effects.
- Drowsy driving can be reduced or ameliorated by addressing chronically short sleep duration and treating sleep disorders.
- Specific countermeasures against drowsy driving can improve driving performance and reduce crash risk.

INTRODUCTION

Drowsy driving occurs when a motor vehicle operator drives while impaired by inadequate or poor sleep, and/or when impaired by a sleepiness-inducing medication or substance. In polls conducted by the National Sleep Foundation, about 60% of drivers admit to driving while feeling sleepy and about 40% have fallen asleep while driving during the previous year.[1,2] Subjective sleepiness while driving is associated with a 2.5-fold increase in the relative risk of a crash.[3] Between 2005 and 2009, an estimated 83,000 crashes occurred each year due to drowsy driving.[4] In 2014 alone, the National Highway Traffic Safety Administration (NHTSA) recorded 846 fatalities directly attributed to drowsy driving, comprising 2.6% of all vehicle crash fatalities.[4] Using additional factors strongly correlated with drowsy driving in the NHTSA's National Automotive Sampling System

Crashworthiness Data System, a study by the AAA Foundation for Traffic Safety estimated that 7% of all crashes and 16.5% of fatal crashes involved drowsy driving, which estimates that more than 5000 people die in fall-asleep crashes in the United States annually.[5]

As discussed in other articles, drowsy driving results from excessive sleepiness identified and quantified by health care providers using a variety of methods and technologies. In this article, we discuss causes of excessive sleepiness while driving amenable to reduction or prevention with appropriate interventions.

PHYSIOLOGY OF DROWSY DRIVING

Excessive sleepiness while driving has many causes, including acute or chronic sleep deprivation, untreated sleep disorders, medical conditions predisposing to fatigue and sleepiness,

a Department of Pulmonary, Critical Care, and Sleep Medicine, VA Puget Sound Health Care System, 1660 South Columbian Way, Seattle, WA 98108, USA; b Department of Psychiatry, University of Washington Sleep Medicine Center, Seattle, WA, USA; c Department of Neurology, University of Washington Sleep Medicine Center, 908 Jefferson Street, Seattle, WA 98104, USA
1 Senior author.
* Corresponding author. Department of Pulmonary, Critical Care, and Sleep Medicine, VA Puget Sound Health Care System, 1660 South Columbian Way, Seattle, WA 98108.
E-mail address: cmccall1@uw.edu

Sleep Med Clin 14 (2019) 469–478
https://doi.org/10.1016/j.jsmc.2019.07.001
1556-407X/19/Published by Elsevier Inc.

sedating medications or substances, and driving at inopportune times in the circadian cycle.[6] These factors are cumulative, with any combination substantially increasing crash risk.[7] Those at highest risk include young male drivers aged 17 to 23 years, individuals with untreated sleep disorders such as obstructive sleep apnea (OSA) and narcolepsy, shift workers, and people sleeping less than 6 hours per night.[4,8]

Sleepy individuals experiencing acute sleep deprivation, chronically short sleep, or poor sleep quality, consistently demonstrate slower reaction times, reduced vigilance, deficits in information processing, and lapses in judgment comparable to driving while legally drunk.[9–12] Sleepy people unknowingly experience "microsleeps," which are brief lapses in consciousness lasting several seconds, accompanied by head nodding, slow eyelid closure, and eyelid drooping.[13,14] Microsleeps lasting 4 to 5 seconds while driving 55 miles per hour mean the driver travels more than 100 yards down the road while asleep. A person's ability to rate their own sleepiness and impairment is negatively impacted by sleepiness, similar to those driving drunk.[15,16]

IDENTIFYING AND TREATING CAUSES OF DROWSY DRIVING

Current society places many demands on adults to meet ever-increasing family, work, and social responsibilities, often at the expense of sleep. This issue is gaining increased awareness within public and private health institutions. The causes of drowsy driving can often be identified and corrected with the appropriate intervention. Several professional societies have published statements urging the implementation of policies to identify and educate those at high risk for fall-asleep crashes on how to recognize and counteract symptoms of drowsy driving.[7,17–20] Numerous studies have investigated the effects of sleep deprivation and sleep disorders on driving safety, as well as improvements in performance with treatment. The following sections detail specific causes of drowsy driving and the benefits of intervention.

Chronic Short Sleep Duration

Industrialized countries face an epidemic of chronic sleep deprivation with many working long hours, commuting long distances, starting school at early hours, caring for family members, and spending increased time using electronic devices during normal sleep hours. Health surveys conducted by the Centers for Disease Control and Prevention report that 35% to 40% of adults in the United States

sleep less than 7 hours per night, and 15% sleep less than 6 hours.[21] This indicates a large proportion of the population sleeps less than the minimum duration of 7 or more hours recommended for all adults by the American Academy of Sleep Medicine and Sleep Research Society.[22] Short sleep duration reduces alertness and performance on vigilance tasks.[23,24] The effects are cumulative such that regularly losing 1 to 2 hours/night creates a "sleep debt" leading to chronic sleepiness in a dose-dependent manner.[15,25–27] Although performance continues to decline with cumulative days of sleep deprivation, subjective ratings of sleepiness level off and drivers are often unaware of their own level of sleepiness.[15,16]

Research demonstrates cognitive benefits with longer sleep, although few studies have investigated whether sleep extension improves driving outcomes. One crossover study examined the effects of sleep extension on psychomotor vigilance task (PVT) performance and daytime sleep latency in adult men before and during total sleep deprivation and after a subsequent recovery sleep. Subjects participated in 2 experimental conditions in a crossover design: habitual sleep (7 hours/night) or extended sleep (average 8.2 hours/night) for 6 nights, followed by "baseline" testing, then a night of total sleep deprivation, and then 10 hours of recovery sleep. After 6 nights of extended sleep, subjects demonstrated improved PVT performance at baseline, during sleep deprivation, and after recovery sleep compared with performance after 6 nights of habitual sleep. Nap latency was also longer at baseline and after recovery sleep for the extended sleep condition compared with the habitual sleep condition.[28] In another study, licensed 16- to 18-year-old drivers regularly sleeping 5 to 7 hours/night underwent 2-week actigraphically monitored periods in which school night bedtimes and rise times were modified to extend time in bed by 1.5 hours/night. Participants reported fewer driving problems during extended sleep periods than during typical sleep periods.[29]

Correcting drowsy driving related to sleep deprivation becomes more complicated when the impaired sleep is related to an untreated sleep disorder, such as OSA.

Obstructive Sleep Apnea

OSA is a sleep disorder whereby repetitive upper airway closures occur during sleep, characterized by snoring and breathing pauses associated with oxygen desaturation and/or cortical arousal. Daytime symptoms associated with OSA include morning headaches, excessive daytime sleepiness (EDS), and low energy. OSA is typically diagnosed with polysomnography (PSG) testing in a laboratory or using a home sleep apnea test. According to the International Classification of Sleep Disorders, 3rd edition, diagnosis of OSA requires an apnea-hypopnea index (AHI) (a measure of breathing pauses or reduced breathing) of at least 15 events per hour, or at least 5 events per hour with symptoms of daytime sleepiness.[30] Approximately 14% of men and 5% of women aged 30 to 70 years meet ICSD-3 diagnostic criteria for OSA.[30,31] The estimated prevalence of OSA in commercial truck drivers is high, ranging from 28% to 80%, likely owing to truck drivers being disproportionately men, middle-aged, and obese.[32,33] Crashes involving commercial vehicles are more likely to result in the death of others on the road, and incur a higher cost.[8,34]

Untreated OSA is associated with increased risk for many chronic health conditions, including hypertension,[35] arrhythmias,[36] myocardial infarction,[37] congestive heart failure,[38] stroke,[39] depression,[40] COPD,[41] type 2 diabetes,[42] and overall mortality.[43] OSA incurs a 2- to 3-fold increased risk of crashes, according to meta-analyses of observational studies.[44,45] Increased risk is associated with body mass index (BMI), AHI, and severity of hypoxemia, but not with self-reported subjective sleepiness.[45] Studies have demonstrated impaired PVT and driver simulator performance in patients with OSA.[46,47] One study showed that in patients with untreated OSA performance was worse on all reaction time measures tested than in those with a blood alcohol concentration of 0.06%.[46] To put this in context, the blood alcohol limit for commercial drivers is 0.04%,[48] with most states enforcing limits between 0.05% and 0.08% for noncommercial drivers.[49]

In recent years, many professional organizations have developed guidelines for identifying, treating, and re-evaluating OSA in commercial drivers.[17,19,28] The American Academy of Sleep Medicine recommends that all transportation workers working in safety-sensitive positions be required to undergo routine screening for OSA.[17] Recommended screening criteria for evaluation by a board-certified sleep medicine specialist include individuals with a BMI $\geq$40, those with fatigue or sleepiness during duty hours or who may have been involved in a drowsy driving crash, and those with a BMI $\geq$35 with either hypertension requiring 2 or more medications, or type 2 diabetes. These criteria are focused on capturing those at highest risk for OSA.[17]

OSA treatment goals are to reduce the AHI to less than 5 events per hour, improve symptoms, and ensure adherence to treatment over time. Several approaches to treating OSA demonstrate varying levels of effectiveness in resolving obstructive respiratory events, reducing daytime sleepiness, and improving driving performance.

Continuous positive airway pressure

The gold standard for treating OSA is continuous positive airway pressure (CPAP) therapy, which delivers pressurized room air through the oronasal cavity to prevent collapse of the upper airway during sleep. PAP therapy has been shown to produce improvement in numerous OSA-associated health conditions, including hypertension,[50,51] cardiovascular events,[52] arrhythmias,[53,54] mortality after stroke,[55] depression,[40] and quality of life.[56]

CPAP therapy significantly reduces subjective and objective measures of sleepiness, such as the Epworth Sleepiness Scale (ESS), the multiple sleep latency test (MSLT), and the maintenance of wakefulness test (MWT).[57–59] In studies assessing impact on drowsy driving, one meta-analysis found a significant risk reduction in motor vehicle crash risk following CPAP treatment (relative risk [RR]= 0.278), with daytime sleepiness improving significantly following a single night of treatment and simulated driving performance improving significantly within 2 to 7 days of CPAP use. OSA treatment lowered crash risk to that of individuals without the disease.[60] Another meta-analysis of CPAP found a significant reduction in real accidents (odds ratio [OR] = 0.21), near-miss accidents (OR = 0.09), and driving simulator accident-related events (standardized mean difference = −1.20) in patients using nasal CPAP.[61]

In commercial drivers, a large-scale, employer-mandated program was conducted for screening, diagnosing, and monitoring OSA adherence in the US trucking industry. Patients with OSA with no adherence to auto-titrating CPAP had a 5-fold greater rate of preventable crashes relative to matched non-OSA controls. The crash rate of patients with OSA with full adherence to CPAP was statistically similar to controls.[62] An employer-driven study at Schneider National found 75% of drivers diagnosed and treated for OSA had a preventable crash during the analysis, with 93% occurring before OSA treatment and 25% occurring after treatment. This represented a 73% reduction in crashes.[63]

Alternative therapies

Although CPAP is considered to be the most effective treatment of OSA, alternative therapies may be considered in those unable to tolerate CPAP. In some individuals, weight loss and/or positional therapy (typically sleeping on one's side or prone) provide enough benefit to effectively prevent obstructive events. Alternative therapies also include oral appliances (OA), which pull the jaw forward during sleep and prevent collapse of soft tissues in the oral airway, or surgical approaches, such as uvulopalatopharyngoplasty (UPPP). Patients with mild OSA are better candidates for OA therapy than those with more severe disease, because of less collapsible airways and greater potential pharyngeal expansion.[64,65] In comparative studies between CPAP and OA treatments, OA is less effective than CPAP for reducing AHI and improving oxygen saturation.[40,64,66,67] However, in some studies, OA has higher compliance than CPAP.[64,68]

Some studies show improvement in simulated driving performance and automobile accidents with alternative therapies.[68,69] After 1 month of CPAP or OA treatment in patients with moderate-severe OSA (mean AHI = 25.6), driving simulator performance improved similarly with both treatment modalities.[68] Although CPAP produced better efficacy in reducing AHI in compliant individuals, OA users exhibited better overall compliance with treatment. Another study found similar simulated driving improvements in both therapeutic modalities after 2 and 3 months.[69] However, given the paucity of long-term data on crash risk reduction or long-term health benefits with OA, the American Academy of Sleep Medicine has not made recommendations regarding the impact of OA on transportation safety.[17,70]

Surgical options for OSA include UPPP, which typically involves the targeted reduction of pharyngeal soft tissues contributing to airway collapse. One study comparing self-reported automobile accident rates between the 5 years before UPPP with the 5 years thereafter found 4 times greater accident risk reduction in UPPP-treated patients than controls, with the relative risk for single-car accidents falling by 83%.[71] This improvement persisted for years after the surgery, although not always in concordance with the residual AHI.[72] Other procedures include temperature-controlled radiofrequency tissue ablation (TCRFTA) to reduce soft tissue volume of the tongue base and palate. One sham-controlled study on TCRFTA found improved subjective sleepiness and reaction time in TCRFTA-treated patients relative to pretreatment baseline, without significant difference between TCRFTA and CPAP.[73] A later study found prolonged improvements in daytime somnolence and psychomotor vigilance at extended follow-up.[73]

Assessing efficacy of therapy
As noted previously, demonstrating effective OSA therapy and reduced drowsy driving risk requires: (a) resolution of obstructive events, (b) adherence

to therapy, and (c) symptom improvement. In the case of PAP therapy, modern PAP devices contain airflow monitoring systems that allow ongoing measurement and reporting of residual obstructive respiratory events. Those treated with OA, positional therapy, significant weight loss, or surgical interventions are recommended to undergo repeat PSG after the intervention to demonstrate adequate resolution of OSA.[17]

Demonstrating adherence to therapy is readily available with PAP devices, which can report the number of days and the average number of h/d the device is used. Current clinical guidelines, and many insurance carriers, consider "adherence" to PAP therapy as using the device at least 4 hours per night on at least 70% of nights during a continuous 30-day period. However, use of PAP therapy for the full duration of sleep provides greater benefits.[17]

When assessing clinical improvement, one must consider whether treatment has improved not only sleepiness, but also vigilance, reaction times, and decision-making processes contributing to fall-asleep crashes. One study assessed subjective sleepiness with the ESS, along with objective neuropsychological tests of alertness, vigilance, driving attention, and driving simulator performance 2 and 42 days after starting CPAP in patients with OSA (mean AHI = 24.8). The study found attention, alertness, accident frequency, and frequency of concentration faults all improved 2 and 42 days after starting CPAP therapy; however, no relationship was found between accident frequency, concentration faults, or subjective daytime sleepiness, and polysomnographic or neuropsychological testing.[74] Another study with 182 patients using CPAP for 1 month with good adherence and adequate therapeutic pressure found improvements in those with mild-moderate and severe OSA in subjective daytime sleepiness, fatigue, and depression, but only patients with severe OSA improved their PVT performance and subjective symptom improvement did not predict PVT performance.[75] Thus clinicians and commercial driver employers should not rely solely on improvements in self-reported sleepiness when assessing drowsy driving risk in patients with OSA.

In addition to reducing sleepiness and improving driving performance, treating OSA reduces costs associated with drowsy driving crashes. One commissioned study by a market research and analytics firm estimated that OSA screening, diagnosis, and treatment saves $1.2 billion for a large trucking company of about 11,000 drivers owing to the high cost of large vehicle accidents.[76]

Hypersomnia Disorders

Hypersomnia disorders are characterized by excessive sleepiness, for which other causes have been ruled out or resolved. In particular, narcolepsy is associated with increased drowsy driving risk owing to frequent unstable sleep-wake transitions typical of this disease.[77] Narcolepsy is characterized by daily periods of irrepressible need to sleep, or daytime lapses into sleep occurring for at least 3 months, with objective measurement of short daytime sleep latency and 2 or more sleep onset rapid eye movement periods during naps on a MSLT.[30] Patients may additionally experience cataplexy, a phenomenon in which strong emotions precipitate a brief (<2 minutes) bilateral loss of muscle tone with retained consciousness. As one might expect, untreated narcolepsy confers elevated risk of fall-asleep crashes. Self-reported driving problems include falling asleep at the wheel, crashes or near crashes from drowsiness or falling asleep, and experiencing cataplexy or sleep paralysis while driving.[78] Those with narcolepsy have a 3- to 4-fold increased risk of crashing, with over one-third reporting an accident because of sleepiness.[78–80] Although crash risk is higher with untreated narcolepsy than untreated OSA, narcolepsy has a much lower prevalence so the absolute number of crashes owing to untreated OSA is much higher.[79]

The mainstay of treatment for hypersomnia disorders is wakefulness-promoting medications.[81] Stimulant medications reduce EDS in patients with narcolepsy.[82,83] However, even with stimulants, the ability of patients with narcolepsy to stay awake is rarely comparable with normal controls.[81,84] The most commonly used agents for residual sleepiness are modafinil and armodafinil, but may also include agents such as methylphenidate or amphetamine salts.[82] Few studies have assessed the efficacy of stimulants on driving performance in narcolepsy patients. One small study with 13 hypersomnia patients found that modafinil improved real driving performance compared with placebo.[85]

Gamma-hydroxybutyrate acid (GHB) also improves sleepiness in narcolepsy. This $GABA_B$ receptor agonist and central nervous system depressant is approved in the form of sodium oxybate (Xyrem) for the treatment of narcolepsy. The medication is taken in 2 doses, one at bedtime and the second 2.5 to 4 hours later. Sodium oxybate was initially indicated for treatment of cataplexy, but also improves subjective daytime sleepiness, increases MWT performance, and reduces sleep attacks in narcoleptic patients.[82,86] The time to treatment response may take as long as 2 months, with 1 study showing the time to maximum response as 106 days for EDS and 213 days for cataplexy.[87] The mechanism for improving EDS is likely because of decreased arousals, increased sleep efficiency, and increased slow-wave sleep as demonstrated on PSG.[88] As a powerful central nervous system depressant, GHB itself can impair driving because of extreme sleepiness, and even "sleep-driving" in patients taking the medication.[89–91] As such, patients should not drive for at least 6 hours after their last dose.[92] However, few studies have assessed the temporal effects of the medication on driving, or the benefits of improved alertness on driving safety. One study assessed the temporal effects of sodium oxybate on driving simulator performance and found severe driving impairment 1 hour after dosing, but no impairment after 3 and 6 hours. Hence safe driving is expected the morning after overnight sodium oxybate use.[89] This is consistent with the rapid clearance and short half-life (30–40 minutes) of the drug.[93]

Some narcolepsy patients obtain alertness benefits from scheduled naps. One study of a repeated nap paradigm in patients with narcolepsy with cataplexy found reaction time performance improved with a single long nap (one-third the duration of nocturnal sleep time) 12 hours after the nocturnal midsleep time.[94]

Stimulant Medications for Excessive Sleepiness

Outside hypersomnia disorder treatment, stimulant medications have narrow indications in select populations following evaluation and treatment of other causes of excessive sleepiness. Stimulant use in patients with chronic short sleep duration or untreated OSA can mask or incompletely resolve physiologic impairment related to sleep deprivation and disruption. One study tested modafinil versus placebo in healthy subjects undergoing 2 nights of total sleep deprivation. The modafinil group experienced fewer lane deviations on a driving simulator test, but did not improve on other measures of driving accuracy such as reaction time, off-road deviations, or speed deviations relative to placebo. Subjects on modafinil also inaccurately rated their own performance as improved relative to placebo.[95]

There are situations in which stimulant medication is appropriate to improve residual sleepiness in patients whose OSA is otherwise effectively treated with CPAP. Treating OSA typically reduces subjective and objective measures of sleepiness.[57,58] However, residual sleepiness can occur in 5% to 55% of CPAP users.[96,97] In patients experiencing EDS with PAP therapy, clinical evaluation is important to identify and resolve other potential contributing factors including: CPAP nonadherence, elevated residual AHI, insufficient nocturnal oxygenation and ventilation, inadequate sleep duration, comorbid sleep disorders, medical conditions, psychiatric illnesses, neurologic diseases, and sedating medication and substance use. In those with residual sleepiness despite resolution of these factors, stimulant medication can increase alertness and reduce drowsy driving risk.[98] One systematic review and meta-analysis of patients with adequate CPAP use receiving pharmacotherapy for residual sleepiness found modafinil and armodafinil improved EDS and attentiveness.[99] However, the effect on driving safety has not been rigorously evaluated.

The benefits of stimulants on clinical symptoms and drowsy driving risk must be weighed against possible adverse treatment effects. Modafinil and armodafinil side effects are generally mild and include headache, nausea, dry mouth, and anorexia.[100] Side effects of stimulant drugs, such as methylphenidate and amphetamine salts include increased anxiety, arrhythmias, anorexia, nausea, insomnia, and psychosis.[101] Abuse potential is problematic in patients receiving stimulant medications, although this problem is rare among individuals with a definitive narcolepsy diagnosis.[82]

Countermeasures for Drowsy Driving

Those with excessive sleepiness because of any cause must be counseled regarding the symptoms and signs of drowsy driving and effective countermeasures. Drowsy driving symptoms include difficulty focusing, daydreaming, disconnected thoughts, heavy eyelids, frequent blinking, yawning, head nodding, lane drifting, and difficulty remembering the last few miles driven.[102,103] The ability to self-rate sleepiness and performance is unreliable.[16] Drivers must plan ahead and not drive when sleepy, keep trips short, or use alternative modes of transportation if sleepiness is anticipated.

Adequate, quality sleep is the only true preventative measure against drowsy driving and fall-asleep crashes. If adequate sleep is not obtained before driving, napping has the greatest positive benefit on performance in sleepy individuals.[104] A short 15- to 20-minute nap improves subsequent performance. Longer naps may produce grogginess.[104–106] Caffeine transiently improves driving performance in sleepy individuals; however, the effect is short, does not address underlying causes of sleepiness, and can mask chronic sleep deprivation.[105,107] Studies show drinking 1 to 2 cups of coffee and pulling over for a 20-minute nap temporarily increases alertness in drowsy drivers.[108] Other countermeasures include brief exercise, listening to music, opening car windows, talking to passengers or on a cell phone, or chewing gum. Evidence is lacking that these are effective countermeasures for drowsy driving, and talking on a cell phone or listening to the radio in fact may increase crash risk.[107,109] Finally, drivers should know alcohol and sedating medications magnify sleepiness and impair driving performance, especially when combined with baseline sleepiness.[110,111] One laboratory-based study found that when individuals were restricted to 4 hours of overnight sleep, 1 unit of beer had the same impact on performance as consuming 6 beers in fully rested individuals.[47]

SUMMARY

Excessive sleepiness while driving is a problem in all industrialized countries and leads to significant morbidity, mortality, and economic cost. The causes of drowsy driving are complex and may be related to chronic insufficient sleep, driving during inopportune times in the circadian cycle, untreated sleep disorders, medical and psychiatric disorders, and use of sedating medication/substances. Those with multiple risk factors are at particularly high risk of drowsy driving and fall-asleep crashes. For example, inexperienced teenage drivers with delayed circadian rhythms and underdeveloped frontal lobes predisposing to impulsive behavior who drive to school for early start times; or sleep-deprived shift workers driving at the sleepiest point in their circadian rhythm; or commercial drivers, with a high prevalence of untreated OSA and extensive time behind the wheel. Identifying and treating these individual problems has in many cases demonstrated improvement in driving performance and reduction of crashes. Although these treatments incur financial cost and lifestyle changes, the benefit in short-term and long-term health and crash reduction are clear. Finally, awareness of countermeasures against drowsy driving must be communicated to anyone at risk of drowsy driving and fall-asleep crashes. Increased provider and public awareness of the need for adequate sleep when operating a motor vehicle is critical for improving the safety of all drivers on public roads.

REFERENCES

1. National Sleep Foundation. Sleep in America Poll 2005: Adult Sleep Habits and Styles. Available

at: https://www.sleepfoundation.org/professionals/sleep-america-polls/2005-adult-sleep-habits-and-styles.

2. Tefft BC. Asleep at the wheel: the prevalence and impact of drowsy driving. Washington, DC: AAA Foundation for Traffic Safety; 2010.

3. Bioulac S, Micoulaud Franchi J-A, Arnaud M, et al. Risk of motor vehicle accidents related to sleepiness at the wheel: a systematic review and meta-analysis. Sleep 2017;40(10). https://doi.org/10.1093/sleep/zsy075.

4. National Highway Traffic Safety Administration. Research on Drowsy Driving. Available at: https://one.nhtsa.gov/Driving-Safety/Drowsy-Driving/Research-on-Drowsy-Driving.

5. Tefft BC. Prevalence of motor vehicle crashes involving drowsy drivers, United States, 1999–2008. Accid Anal Prev 2012;45:180–6.

6. Wheaton AG, Shults RA, Chapman DP, et al, Division of Population Health, National Center for Chronic Disease Prevention and Health Promotion. Drowsy driving and risk behaviors - 10 States and Puerto Rico, 2011-2012. MMWR Morb Mortal Wkly Rep 2014;63(26):557–62.

7. NCSDR/NHTSA Expert Panel on Driver Fatigue and Sleepiness. Drowsy Driving and Automobile Crashes. Available at: https://www.nhlbi.nih.gov/files/docs/resources/sleep/drsy_drv.pdf.

8. National Highway Safety Traffic Administration, US Department of Transportation. Traffic Safety Facts 2014. Available at: https://crashstats.nhtsa.dot.gov/Api/Public/Publication/812261.

9. Lim J, Dinges DF. Sleep deprivation and vigilant attention. Ann N Y Acad Sci 2008;1129(1):305–22.

10. Dawson D, Reid K. Fatigue, alcohol and performance impairment. Nature 1997;388(6639):235.

11. Powell NB, Schechtman KB, Riley RW, et al. The road to danger: the comparative risks of driving while sleepy. Laryngoscope 2001;111(5):887–93.

12. Williamson AM, Feyer AM. Moderate sleep deprivation produces impairments in cognitive and motor performance equivalent to legally prescribed levels of alcohol intoxication. Occup Environ Med 2000; 57(10):649–55.

13. Durmer JS, Dinges DF. Neurocognitive consequences of sleep deprivation. Semin Neurol 2005; 25(01):117–29.

14. Alvaro PK, Jackson ML, Berlowitz DJ, et al. Prolonged eyelid closure episodes during sleep deprivation in professional drivers. J Clin Sleep Med 2016;12(8):1099–103.

15. Van Dongen HPA, Maislin G, Mullington JM, et al. The cumulative cost of additional wakefulness: dose-response effects on neurobehavioral functions and sleep physiology from chronic sleep restriction and total sleep deprivation. Sleep 2003; 26(2):117–26.

16. Reyner LA, Horne JA. Falling asleep whilst driving: are drivers aware of prior sleepiness? Int J Legal Med 1998;111(3):120–3.

17. Gurubhagavatula I, Sullivan S, Meoli A, et al. Management of obstructive sleep apnea in commercial motor vehicle operators: recommendations of the AASM sleep and transportation safety awareness task force. J Clin Sleep Med 2017;13(05):745–58.

18. Higgins JS, Michael J, Austin R, et al. Asleep at the wheel—the road to addressing drowsy driving. Sleep 2017;40(2).

19. Mukherjee S, Patel SR, Kales SN, et al. An official American Thoracic Society statement: the importance of healthy sleep. Recommendations and future priorities. Am J Respir Crit Care Med 2015; 191(12):1450–8.

20. National Research Council (US), Institute of Medicine (US), Transportation Research Board (US) Program Committee for a workshop on contributions from the behavioral and social sciences in reducing and preventing teen motor crashes. Preventing teen motor crashes: contributions from the behavioral and social sciences: workshop report. Washington, DC: National Academies Press; 2007.

21. Centers for Disease Control and Prevention (CDC). Effect of short sleep duration on daily activities–United States, 2005-2008. MMWR Morb Mortal Wkly Rep 2011;60(8):239–42.

22. Watson NF, Badr MS, Belenky G, et al. Joint consensus statement of the American Academy of Sleep Medicine and Sleep Research Society on the recommended amount of sleep for a healthy adult: methodology and discussion. Sleep 2015; 38(8):1161–83.

23. Rosenthal L, Roehrs TA, Rosen A, et al. Level of sleepiness and total sleep time following various time in bed conditions. Sleep 1993;16(3):226–32.

24. Goel N, Rao H, Durmer JS, et al. Neurocognitive consequences of sleep deprivation. Semin Neurol 2009;29(4):320–39.

25. Carskadon MA, Dement WC. Cumulative effects of sleep restriction on daytime sleepiness. Psychophysiology 1981;18(2):107–13.

26. Dinges DF, Pack F, Williams K, et al. Cumulative sleepiness, mood disturbance, and psychomotor vigilance performance decrements during a week of sleep restricted to 4-5 hours per night. Sleep 1997;20(4):267–77.

27. Belenky G, Wesensten NJ, Thorne DR, et al. Patterns of performance degradation and restoration during sleep restriction and subsequent recovery: a sleep dose-response study. J Sleep Res 2003; 12(1):1–12.

28. Arnal PJ, Sauvet F, Leger D, et al. Benefits of sleep extension on sustained attention and sleep

pressure before and during total sleep deprivation and recovery. Sleep 2015;38(12):1935–43.

29. Garner AA, Hansen A, Baxley C, et al. Effect of sleep extension on sluggish cognitive tempo symptoms and driving behavior in adolescents with chronic short sleep. Sleep Med 2017;30:93–6.

30. American Academy of Sleep Medicine. The International Classification of sleep disorders - third Edition (ICSD-3). Darien (IL): American Academy of Sleep Medicine; 2014.

31. Peppard PE, Young T, Barnet JH, et al. Increased prevalence of sleep-disordered breathing in adults. Am J Epidemiol 2013;177(9):1006–14.

32. Howard ME, Desai AV, Grunstein RR, et al. Sleepiness, sleep-disordered breathing, and accident risk factors in commercial vehicle drivers. Am J Respir Crit Care Med 2004;170(9):1014–21.

33. Stoohs RA, Bingham LA, Itoi A, et al. Sleep and sleep-disordered breathing in commercial long-haul truck drivers. Chest 1995;107(5):1275–82.

34. Zaloshnja E., Miller T. Revised costs of large truck- and bus-involved crashes, 2002. Washington, DC: U.S. Department of Transportation, Federal Motor Carrier Safety Administration. Available at: https://www.fmcsa.dot.gov/sites/fmcsa.dot.gov/files/docs/RevisedCostLargeTruckBusCrashes2002.pdf.

35. Nieto FJ, Young TB, Lind BK, et al. Association of sleep-disordered breathing, sleep apnea, and hypertension in a large community-based study. Sleep Heart Health Study. JAMA 2000;283(14):1829–36.

36. Digby GC, Baranchuk A. Sleep apnea and atrial fibrillation; 2012 update. Curr Cardiol Rev 2012;8(4):265–72.

37. Hung J, Whitford EG, Parsons RW, et al. Association of sleep apnoea with myocardial infarction in men. Lancet 1990;336(8710):261–4.

38. Oldenburg O, Lamp B, Faber L, et al. Sleep-disordered breathing in patients with symptomatic heart failure: a contemporary study of prevalence in and characteristics of 700 patients. Eur J Heart Fail 2007;9(3):251–7.

39. Dyken ME, Im K. Obstructive sleep apnea and stroke. Chest 2009;136(6):1668–77.

40. Gagnadoux F, Le Vaillant M, Goupil F, et al. Depressive symptoms before and after long-term CPAP therapy in patients with sleep apnea. Chest 2014;145(5):1025–31.

41. Romem A, Iacono A, McIlmoyle E, et al. Obstructive sleep apnea in patients with end-stage lung disease. J Clin Sleep Med 2013;9(7):687–93.

42. Foster GD, Sanders MH, Millman R, et al. Obstructive sleep apnea among obese patients with type 2 diabetes. Diabetes Care 2009;32(6):1017–9.

43. Punjabi NM, Caffo BS, Goodwin JL, et al. Sleep-disordered breathing and mortality: a prospective cohort study. PLoS Med 2009;6(8):e1000132.

44. Strohl KP, Brown DB, Collop N, et al. An official American Thoracic Society clinical practice guideline: sleep apnea, sleepiness, and driving risk in noncommercial drivers. An update of a 1994 statement. Am J Respir Crit Care Med 2013;187(11):1259–66.

45. Tregear S, Reston J, Schoelles K, et al. Obstructive sleep apnea and risk of motor vehicle crash: systematic review and meta-analysis. J Clin Sleep Med 2009;5(6):573–81.

46. Powell NB, Riley RW, Schechtman KB, et al. A comparative model: reaction time performance in sleep-disordered breathing versus alcohol-impaired controls. Laryngoscope 1999;109(10):1648–54.

47. Roehrs T, Beare D, Zorick F, et al. Sleepiness and ethanol effects on simulated driving. Alcohol Clin Exp Res 1994;18(1):154–8.

48. Federal Motor Carrier Safety Administration D of T. Section A § 382.201 - Alcohol Concentration. Title 49 - Transportation. Subtitle B - Other Regulations Relating to Transportation (Continued). Federal Motor Carrier Safety Regulations.; 2006.

49. National Conference of State Legislatures. Drunken Driving. Available at: http://www.ncsl.org/research/transportation/drunken-driving.aspx.

50. Duran-Cantolla J, Aizpuru F, Montserrat JM, et al. Continuous positive airway pressure as treatment for systemic hypertension in people with obstructive sleep apnoea: randomised controlled trial. BMJ 2010;341(nov24 1):c5991.

51. Martínez-García M-A, Capote F, Campos-Rodríguez F, et al. Effect of CPAP on blood pressure in patients with obstructive sleep apnea and resistant hypertension. JAMA 2013;310(22):2407.

52. Marin JM, Carrizo SJ, Vicente E, et al. Long-term cardiovascular outcomes in men with obstructive sleep apnoea-hypopnoea with or without treatment with continuous positive airway pressure: an observational study. Lancet 2005;365(9464):1046–53.

53. Kanagala R, Murali NS, Friedman PA, et al. Obstructive sleep apnea and the recurrence of atrial fibrillation. Circulation 2003;107(20):2589–94.

54. Fein AS, Shvilkin A, Shah D, et al. Treatment of obstructive sleep apnea reduces the risk of atrial fibrillation recurrence after catheter ablation. J Am Coll Cardiol 2013;62(4):300–5.

55. Martínez-García MÁ, Soler-Cataluña JJ, Ejarque-Martínez L, et al. Continuous positive airway pressure treatment reduces mortality in patients with ischemic stroke and obstructive sleep apnea. Am J Respir Crit Care Med 2009;180(1):36–41.

56. Bolitschek J, Schmeiser-Rieder A, Schobersberger R, et al. Impact of nasal continuous positive airway pressure treatment on quality of life in patients with obstructive sleep apnoea. Eur Respir J 1998;11(4):890–4.

57. Patel SR, White DP, Malhotra A, et al. Continuous positive airway pressure therapy for treating sleepiness in a diverse population with obstructive sleep apnea: results of a meta-analysis. Arch Intern Med 2003;163(5):565–71.

58. Marshall NS, Barnes M, Travier N, et al. Continuous positive airway pressure reduces daytime sleepiness in mild to moderate obstructive sleep apnoea: a meta-analysis. Thorax 2006;61(5):430–4.

59. Zhao YY, Wang R, Gleason KJ, et al. Effect of continuous positive airway pressure treatment on health-related quality of life and sleepiness in high cardiovascular risk individuals with sleep apnea: best apnea interventions for research (BestAIR) trial. Sleep 2017;40(4). https://doi.org/10.1093/sleep/zsx040.

60. Tregear S, Reston J, Schoelles K, et al. Continuous positive airway pressure reduces risk of motor vehicle crash among drivers with obstructive sleep apnea: systematic review and meta-analysis. Sleep 2010;33(10):1373–80.

61. Antonopoulos CN, Sergentanis TN, Daskalopoulou SS, et al. Nasal continuous positive airway pressure (nCPAP) treatment for obstructive sleep apnea, road traffic accidents and driving simulator performance: a meta-analysis. Sleep Med Rev 2011;15(5):301–10.

62. Burks SV, Anderson JE, Bombyk M, et al. Nonadherence with employer-mandated sleep apnea treatment and increased risk of serious truck crashes. Sleep 2016;39(5):967–75.

63. Berger M, Sullivan W, R O, Wu C. USAA Corporate-Driven Sleep Apnea Detection and Treatment Program: Results and Challenges. https://pdfs.semanticscholar.org/0ebd/2ba29b10c54fffe1331935715693caeee5f9.pdf.

64. Marklund M. Update on oral appliance therapy for OSA. Curr Sleep Med Rep 2017;3(3):143–51.

65. Edwards BA, Andara C, Landry S, et al. Upper-airway collapsibility and loop gain predict the response to oral appliance therapy in patients with obstructive sleep apnea. Am J Respir Crit Care Med 2016;194(11):1413–22.

66. Barnes M, McEvoy RD, Banks S, et al. Efficacy of positive airway pressure and oral appliance in mild to moderate obstructive sleep apnea. Am J Respir Crit Care Med 2004;170(6):656–64.

67. Lam B, Sam K, Mok WY, et al. Randomised study of three non-surgical treatments in mild to moderate obstructive sleep apnoea. Thorax 2007;62(4):354–9.

68. Phillips CL, Grunstein RR, Darendeliler MA, et al. Health outcomes of continuous positive airway pressure versus oral appliance treatment for obstructive sleep apnea. Am J Respir Crit Care Med 2013;187(8):879–87.

69. Hoekema A, Stegenga B, Bakker M, et al. Simulated driving in obstructive sleep apnoea-hypopnoea; effects of oral appliances and continuous positive airway pressure. Sleep Breath 2007;11(3):129–38.

70. American Academy of Sleep Medicine. Response to the advance Notice of Proposed Rulemaking regarding the evaluation of safety sensitive Personnel for moderate-to-severe obstructive sleep apnea. Available at: https://aasm.org/resources/pdf/government/fmcsa-fra-response-aasm.pdf.

71. Haraldsson PO, Carenfelt C, Lysdahl M, et al. Does uvulopalatopharyngoplasty inhibit automobile accidents? Laryngoscope 1995;105(6):657–61.

72. Haraldsson PO, Carenfelt C, Lysdahl M, et al. Long-term effect of uvulopalatopharyngoplasty on driving performance. Arch Otolaryngol Head Neck Surg 1995;121(1):90–4.

73. Woodson BT, Steward DL, Weaver EM, et al. A randomized trial of temperature-controlled radiofrequency, continuous positive airway pressure, and placebo for obstructive sleep apnea syndrome. Otolaryngol Head Neck Surg 2003;128(6):848–61.

74. Orth M, Duchna H-W, Leidag M, et al. Driving simulator and neuropyschological testing in OSAS before and under CPAP therapy. Eur Respir J 2005;26(5):898–903.

75. Bhat S, Gupta D, Akel O, et al. The relationships between improvements in daytime sleepiness, fatigue and depression and psychomotor vigilance task testing with CPAP use in patients with obstructive sleep apnea. Sleep Med 2018;49:81–9.

76. Frost & Sullivan. Hidden health crisis costing America billions: underdiagnosing and undertreating obstructive sleep apnea draining healthcare system. Darien (IL): American Academy of Sleep Medicine; 2016.

77. Liu S-Y, Perez MA, Lau N. The impact of sleep disorders on driving safety—findings from the Second Strategic Highway Research Program naturalistic driving study. Sleep 2018;41(4). https://doi.org/10.1093/sleep/zsy023.

78. Valley V, Broughton R. Daytime performance deficits and physiological vigilance in untreated patients with narcolepsy-cataplexy compared to controls. Rev Electroencephalogr Neurophysiol Clin 1981;11(1):133–9.

79. Aldrich MS. Automobile accidents in patients with sleep disorders. Sleep 1989;12(6):487–94.

80. Pizza F, Jaussent I, Lopez R, et al. Car crashes and central disorders of hypersomnolence: a French study. PLoS One 2015;10(6):e0129386.

81. Mitler MM, Aldrich MS, Koob GF, et al. Narcolepsy and its treatment with stimulants. ASDA standards of practice. Sleep 1994;17(4):352–71.

82. Takenoshita S, Nishino S. Pharmacologic management of excessive daytime sleepiness. Sleep Med Clin 2017;12(3):461–78.

83. US Modafinil in Narcolepsy Multicenter Study Group. Randomized trial of modafinil as a treatment for the excessive daytime somnolence of narcolepsy. Neurology 2000;54(5):1166–75.

84. Boivin DB, Montplaisir J, Petit D, et al. Effects of modafinil on symptomatology of human narcolepsy. Clin Neuropharmacol 1993;16(1):46–53.

85. Philip P, Chaufton C, Taillard J, et al. Modafinil improves real driving performance in patients with hypersomnia: a randomized double-blind placebo-controlled crossover clinical trial. Sleep 2014; 37(3):483–7.

86. Alshaikh MK, Tricco AC, Tashkandi M, et al. Sodium oxybate for narcolepsy with cataplexy: systematic review and meta-analysis. J Clin Sleep Med 2012; 8(4):451–8.

87. Bogan RK, Roth T, Schwartz J, et al. Time to response with sodium oxybate for the treatment of excessive daytime sleepiness and cataplexy in patients with narcolepsy. J Clin Sleep Med 2015; 11(4):427–32.

88. Plazzi G, Pizza F, Vandi S, et al. Impact of acute administration of sodium oxybate on nocturnal sleep polysomnography and on multiple sleep latency test in narcolepsy with cataplexy. Sleep Med 2014;15(9):1046–54.

89. Liakoni E, Dempsey DA, Meyers M, et al. Effect of γ-hydroxybutyrate (GHB) on driving as measured by a driving simulator. Psychopharmacology (Berl) 2018;235(11):3223–32.

90. Centola C, Giorgetti A, Zaami S, et al. Effects of GHB on psychomotor and driving performance. Curr Drug Metab 2018;19(13):1065–72.

91. Wallace DM, Maze T, Shafazand S. Sodium oxybate-induced sleep driving and sleep-related eating disorder. J Clin Sleep Med 2011;7(3):310–1.

92. Jazz Pharmaceuticals. Taking Xyrem. Available at: https://www.xyrem.com/xyrem-dosing-narcolepsy-cataplexy-eds.

93. Liechti ME, Quednow BB, Liakoni E, et al. Pharmacokinetics and pharmacodynamics of γ-hydroxybutyrate in healthy subjects. Br J Clin Pharmacol 2016;81(5):980–8.

94. Mullington J, Broughton R. Scheduled naps in the management of daytime sleepiness in narcolepsy-cataplexy. Sleep 1993;16(5):444–56.

95. Gurtman CG, Broadbear JH, Redman JR. Effects of modafinil on simulator driving and self-assessment of driving following sleep deprivation. Hum Psychopharmacol 2008;23(8):681–92.

96. Gasa M, Tamisier R, Launois SH, et al. Residual sleepiness in sleep apnea patients treated by continuous positive airway pressure. J Sleep Res 2013;22(4):389–97.

97. Koutsourelakis I, Perraki E, Economou NT, et al. Predictors of residual sleepiness in adequately treated obstructive sleep apnoea patients. Eur Respir J 2009;34(3):687–93.

98. Chapman JL, Serinel Y, Marshall NS, et al. Residual daytime sleepiness in obstructive sleep apnea after continuous positive airway pressure optimization. Sleep Med Clin 2016;11(3):353–63.

99. Avellar ABCC, Carvalho LBC, Prado GF, et al. Pharmacotherapy for residual excessive sleepiness and cognition in CPAP-treated patients with obstructive sleep apnea syndrome: a systematic review and meta-analysis. Sleep Med Rev 2016; 30:97–107.

100. Roth T, Schwartz JRL, Hirshkowitz M, et al. Evaluation of the safety of modafinil for treatment of excessive sleepiness. J Clin Sleep Med 2007; 3(6):595–602.

101. Leonard BE, McCartan D, White J, et al. Methylphenidate: a review of its neuropharmacological, neuropsychological and adverse clinical effects. Hum Psychopharmacol 2004;19(3):151–80.

102. Lyznicki JM, Doege TC, Davis RM, et al. Sleepiness, driving, and motor vehicle crashes. Council on Scientific Affairs, American Medical Association. JAMA 1998;279(23):1908–13.

103. Mathis J, Hess CW. Sleepiness and vigilance tests. Swiss Med Wkly 2009;139(15–16):214–9.

104. Dinges DF, Orne MT, Whitehouse WG, et al. Temporal placement of a nap for alertness: contributions of circadian phase and prior wakefulness. Sleep 1987;10(4):313–29.

105. Spaeth AM, Goel N, Dinges DF. Cumulative neurobehavioral and physiological effects of chronic caffeine intake: individual differences and implications for the use of caffeinated energy products. Nutr Rev 2014;72(Suppl 1):34–47.

106. Wertz AT, Ronda JM, Czeisler CA, et al. Effects of sleep inertia on cognition. JAMA 2006;295(2):163–4.

107. Horne JA, Reyner LA. Driver sleepiness. J Sleep Res 1995;4(S2):23–9.

108. Reyner LA, Horne JA. Suppression of sleepiness in drivers: combination of caffeine with a short nap. Psychophysiology 1997;34(6):721–5.

109. Redelmeier DA, Tibshirani RJ. Association between cellular-telephone calls and motor vehicle collisions. N Engl J Med 1997;336(7):453–8.

110. Wilkinson RT, Colquhoun WP. Interaction of alcohol with incentive and with sleep deprivation. J Exp Psychol 1968;76(4):623–9.

111. Dassanayake T, Michie P, Carter G, et al. Effects of benzodiazepines, antidepressants and opioids on driving. Drug Saf 2011;34(2):125–56.

Vehicle and Highway Adaptations to Compensate for Sleepy Drivers

Mark E. Howard, MBBS, PhD[a,b,c,*], Jennifer M. Cori, PhD[a],
William J. Horrey, PhD[d]

KEYWORDS

- Sleepiness • Automobile driving • Traffic accidents • Advanced driver assistance systems
- Drowsiness monitoring • Roadside barrier • Rumble strip

KEY POINTS

- Eliminating sleepiness-related road crashes is challenging given the high prevalence of sleep disorders and shift work, with vehicle and road safety adaptations important pillars in creating a safe road system.
- Continuous driver monitoring using physiologic measures, such as slowing of eyelid movements, and changes in driver behavior, including altered steering responses, can identify sleepy drivers and prompt early interventions.
- Vehicle adaptations now enable early warning of lane drafting and hazards with emerging automated technology taking control of the vehicle in some emergencies. As autonomous vehicles develop, technology will need to determine that the driver is alert and able to resume vehicle control.
- Road adaptations that alert drivers to lane departure (rumble strips) and prevent run off road incidents (flexible roadside barriers) substantially reduce the frequency and severity of run off the road crashes that are frequently sleepiness related.

INTRODUCTION

Leading road safety countries have evolved a "Safe System" approach to addressing the risk of crashes, injury, and mortality. The underlying philosophy accepts that road users will inevitably make mistakes that can lead to harm and that there is a shared responsibility for designers and builders of roads and vehicles to minimize risk in addition to the responsibility of drivers.[1] The key pillars of this system have been considered as safe roads, speeds, vehicles, and road users. These are general principles irrespective of the cause of road crashes that equally apply to sleepy driving. Respecting the latter, it is important to minimize the risk of sleepy driving through

Disclosure Statement: M.E. Howard is a Theme Leader in the Co-operative Research Center for Alertness, Safety and Productivity and received equipment support for research from Optalert, Seeing Machines and SmartCap. J.M. Cori receives research funding from the Co-operative Research Center for Alertness, Safety and Productivity and has received equipment support for research from Optalert and Seeing Machines. W.J. Horrey has no conflicts of interest.

[a] Institute for Breathing and Sleep, Austin Health, 145 Studley Road, Heidelberg, Victoria 3084, Australia; [b] University of Melbourne, Parkville, Victoria, Australia; [c] School of Psychological Sciences, Monash University, Clayton, Victoria, Australia; [d] Traffic Research Group, AAA Foundation for Traffic Safety, 607 14th Street Northwest, Suite 201, Washington, DC 20005, USA
* Corresponding author. Institute for Breathing and Sleep, Austin Health, 145 Studley Road, Heidelberg, Victoria 3084, Australia.
E-mail address: Mark.howard@austin.org.au

Sleep Med Clin 14 (2019) 479–489
https://doi.org/10.1016/j.jsmc.2019.08.005
1556-407X/19/© 2019 Elsevier Inc. All rights reserved.

managing sleep disorders, optimizing schedules for shift workers, and public education. However, although these efforts might help reduce the prevalence, they will not eradicate sleepy driving. For example, shift workers driving home after night shift, truck drivers driving at night, and those with undiagnosed sleep disorders will remain at risk. As such, road infrastructure and vehicle countermeasures to help reduce or mitigate the risks of sleepy driving are needed.

Analysis of fatal crashes in Sweden suggested that road design was the largest individual contributor, followed by the driver and then vehicle standards.[2,3] It was estimated that 90% of fatalities would have been preventable by good road design, 55% by optimal road user compliance, and 34% by improved vehicle design. Hence, vehicle and road construction initiatives that assist with mitigating risk are important for minimizing the impact of sleepy driving crashes. The current article reviews and highlights a range of these established and evolving innovations and initiatives.

Physiologic and Behavioral Sleepiness Indicators: Targets for Intervention

Although the subjective experience of sleepiness varies across individuals, there are a number of observable physiologic changes that occur with increasing sleepiness. These progressive changes occur irrespective of whether this is secondary to a sleep disorder, sleep restriction, or circadian rhythm effects. Slowing of electrical activity in the brain on electroencephalogram (EEG) occurs in conjunction with slowing of eye and eye lid movements, reduced visual scanning, and longer reaction times (**Fig. 1**).[4,5] This results in abnormal driver behavior, including greater variation in speed and lane position, episodes of drifting out of the lane, slower breaking reaction time, failure to detect hazards and road signage, and potentially fall asleep events with run off the road crashes (see **Fig. 1**).[4–6] To the extent that they can provide ample warning before a crash or a safety critical event, these indicators, both physiologic measures derived from the driver and measures of driving performance, provide potential targets for vehicle and road/highway adaptations to prevent crashes or at least mitigate the effect of crashes.

VEHICLE SAFETY ADAPTATIONS
Direct Drowsiness Monitoring via Physiologic Metrics

Drowsiness is associated with changes in physiologic metrics that can be measured continuously during driving. Eye blink–related parameters and brain activity, measured by EEG, are the most commonly assessed physiologic indicators of drowsiness. Eye blink parameters are monitored either via a camera mounted to the vehicle or sensors attached to the face or accessories worn by the driver. Moderate-strength correlations have been observed between eye blink measures of drowsiness and driving performance metrics of lane position, speed, crash occurrence, and reaction times. Eye blink parameters, particularly blink duration, also predict on road out of lane events[4,5,7,8] and self-rated sleep and inattention driving events.[9] Several driver drowsiness monitoring devices are based on these measures. Optalert comprises an infrared sensor embedded within a glasses frame.[10] It uses several eye blink parameters in a proprietary algorithm and alerts the driver when a critical threshold is exceeded,[10] which has been shown to reduce eye blink measures of drowsiness by approximately 20%.[11] Similar findings have been observed for the Seeing Machines commercial driver system, which detects eye closure. In a single company that used Seeing Machines from 2011 to 2016, the incidence of fatigue scored events (eye closures >1.5 seconds) decreased by 66% when driver feedback was on and by 95% when the feedback was additionally provided to the employer.[12]

EEG is traditionally considered the gold standard for assessing alertness state.[13] In simulated driving and on road studies there is slowing of EEG activity and increased microsleeps at night and following sleep restriction, with time on task effects also observed.[6,14,15] EEG monitoring during driving has been technically difficult due to signal noise and inability to conduct real-time analysis. However, wireless commercial devices have emerged.[16] SmartCap provides online EEG monitoring and drowsiness warning via electrodes that are embedded within a regular cap or safety cap. Although there are limited data evaluating SmartCap, a laboratory report found that it detects severe sleepiness well,[16] and in a field study the signal varied consistently with expected circadian variation.[17]

Indirect Drowsiness Monitoring via Vehicle Performance Metrics

As drowsiness increases, the ability of drivers to maintain effective vehicle control deteriorates. Thus, vehicle performance metrics provide an indirect measure of drowsiness. Steering wheel movement, brake force, and speed maintenance have been evaluated for drowsiness monitoring in the

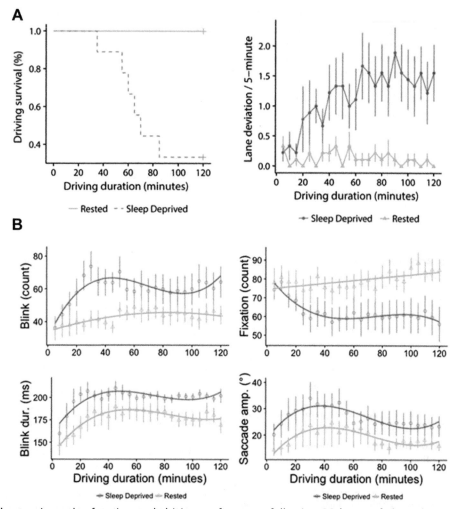

Fig. 1. Changes in ocular function and driving performance following 36 hours of sleep deprivation (*red*) compared with controls (*green*) during real driving. (*A*) Kaplan-Meier curve for drive terminations and number of lane departure events per 5-minute block of driving with standard error. (*B*) Mean and standard error with curvilinear fit for blink rate, blink duration, fixation rate, and saccade amplitude. (*From* Shiferaw BA, Downey LA, Westlake J, et al. Stationary gaze entropy predicts lane departure events in sleep-deprived drivers. *Sci Rep.* 2018;8(1):2220; with permission.)

laboratory and field; however, only steering wheel movement has been implemented as a key component in commercial devices.

Steering wheel movement is typically measured via steering wheel angle but also can be inferred from the standard deviation of lateral position (SDLP) of a vehicle within a lane. Alert drivers make frequent but small steering wheel corrections to maintain lane position, whereas sleep-deprived drivers make infrequent but large magnitude corrections and have greater SDLP.[15,18,19] Real on road driving data from the Mercedes Benz Drowsiness Database supports these findings, with greater velocity of steering wheel corrections observed when drivers' self-rate as drowsy.[20] Mercedes Benz has incorporated steering wheel movement into their drive attention-assist system available in some car models. There is also a commercial after-market device available, the Advisory System for Tired Drivers (ASTiD), that relies on steering wheel adjustments to help inform fatigue levels, although this system also uses metrics that are not related to vehicle performance, such as prior sleep quality, circadian time of day, and driving distance.[21]

Comparison of Indirect Vehicle Performance Versus Direct Physiologic Measures

As physiologic metrics provide a direct measure of drowsiness state, they may provide an earlier indication of alertness failure than vehicle performance metrics. Another advantage of physiologic metrics is that they are less affected by factors unrelated to drowsiness, such as environment (weather, temperature, and lighting), driver characteristics (driver experience and attitude), road conditions (traffic, speed, lane markings), and vehicle specifications. Physiologic metrics can be considered obtrusive and less acceptable to drivers than vehicle performance metrics.[22] As technology advances, this should improve; however, a recent review highlighted that currently many of the physiologic drowsiness monitoring devices lack complete and independent validation studies (**Table 1** details of common commercially available systems).[10]

Drowsiness Monitoring System Implementation and Implications

The ultimate goal of drowsiness monitoring systems is to alert the driver and potentially company when vehicle performance or physiologic metrics exceed a threshold associated with an unsafe level of drowsiness. Feedback is typically a combination of auditory or visual stimuli that provide an alert to the driver when levels are unsafe. Preliminary field research suggests that drivers have increased physiologic alertness using these systems with the feedback on.[11] Whether this is a direct effect of the alert or a result of drivers actively adjusting their behavior as a result of being monitored (eg, increasing habitual sleep duration, having naps, or increasing caffeine), is unknown. Further work in larger samples is required to determine how alertness is improved and if the effect is long lasting.

General Vehicle Adaptations

In addition to technologies that monitor driver state and drowsiness, other active and passive vehicle systems can help avoid crashes or reduce the severity of crashes. These systems stand to benefit all drivers, not only sleepy ones, and range from systems that warn drivers of impending collisions to highly automated systems, in which the vehicle itself takes on more of the driving responsibilities.

Forward collision warning (FCW) and automatic emergency braking (AEB) systems use sensor technologies to detect when a crash is imminent. FCW provides an alert to drivers, ideally affording them sufficient time to orient, plan, and execute an appropriate avoidance maneuver. AEB systems automatically apply the vehicle's brakes to avoid or reduce the severity of a crash with on object in front of the vehicle. Typically, AEB operates

on a shorter timeframe than FCW and, in many cases, systems provide a warning in advance of automatic braking. Several studies have identified the potential for these systems to address a significant number of motor vehicle crashes, injuries, and fatalities in the United States[23,24] or actual reduction in crash-related insurance claims.[25] For example, Benson and colleagues[26] estimated that these systems, if installed on all passenger vehicles, would theoretically prevent upward of 29% of all crashes and 14% of fatal crashes.

With respect to drowsy drivers, Gaspar and colleagues[27] found that FCW was effective at reducing response times to critical events in moderately and severely fatigued drivers, but only when the driver's gaze was initially off-road (at the time of the alert). This suggests that these systems might be effective at helping drowsy drivers reorient toward the forward roadway; however, more work is needed to understand the dependencies of FCW benefits and initial gaze location. AEB systems offer further benefits and protections for drowsy drivers, as these systems automatically execute the emergency maneuver, without requiring that the driver fully orient themselves, and select and execute a course of action.

Lane departure warning (LDW) and lane keeping assist (LKA) systems use on-board sensors and/or cameras to track the vehicles' position within the lane boundaries. When the system detects an unintentional lane departure, typically indicated by the absence of the turn indicator, then an alert is issued. LKA systems will automatically steer the vehicle back toward the center of the lane to prevent the departure. It is estimated that these technologies could help mitigate 7% of all crashes and 14% of fatal crashes in the United States.[26,28] Although these analyses did not focus on the benefits for drowsy drivers, the crash configurations that these systems aim to prevent map onto those commonly associated with drowsy driving (eg, single-vehicle crashes, run off road, head-on crashes[29]). Response times to lane departure events and corrective maneuvers have improved in simulator studies of LDW in drowsy drivers.[30]

Importantly, providing warnings to drivers, especially those who are drowsy or already asleep, might not always help them avoid a crash. Active crash avoidance systems such as AEB and LKA offer enhanced safety benefits; however, automated driving systems that take on more of the driving responsibilities under normal operating conditions are becoming more commonplace. For example, these systems can adjust the vehicle speed to maintain a preferred spacing with a lead vehicle (eg, adaptive cruise control) or can actively steer the vehicle to keep the vehicle in

Table 1
Vehicle and physiologic measures of drowsiness designed for use in vehicle

Drowsiness Measure	Device	Method	Output	Laboratory and/or Field Support
Steering wheel movement	ASTiD	• Gyroscopes detect rate of steering wheel turn and exaggerated corrections. • This is combined with time of day, driver sleep quality input and drive length and type.	• Fatigue index is updated each minute and is displayed on a dashboard-mounted device. • Real-time auditory and visual alerts are provided to the driver and central dispatch operators.	Field: • Trialed in the mining sector with more than 1000 hours of use and received positive feedback, with uses reported that the system typically reflected how they were feeling, but some reported alerts when they were not sleepy at all[70]
Eye-related monitoring	Optalert	• Measures the velocity and amplitude of the eyelid opening and closing using an infrared sensor built into a glasses frame that can be worn with prescription lenses.	• Johns Drowsiness Score (JDS) is updated each minute and displayed on a device. • JDS ranges from 0 (very alert) to 10 (very drowsy) and provides alerts to drivers when scores reach critical levels. • JDS can also be relayed to managers in real-time.	Laboratory: • Predicts subjective sleepiness[68] • Predicts neurobehavioral and simulated driving task performance[18,68,69] Field: • Associated with inattention and sleep-related driving events.[9] • Increases significantly following night shift drives compared with alert drives.[6,9] • Improves alertness by 20% when feedback is on[11]
	Seeing Machines Guardian	• Video camera combined with face and gaze tracking algorithms detect drowsiness-related events based on eye closure and head position. • Events are wirelessly uploaded and validated centrally by a trained observer.	• An auditory verbal warning/tone and seat vibration occurs if a fatigue event has been detected. • Alerts also can be provided to operators.	Field: • Commercial truck fleet data from a single company in 2011–2016 found a 66% reduction in fatigue events with driver feedback on and a 95% reduction with the addition of operator feedback.[12]
Brain wave monitoring	Smart Cap	• Measures EEG via electrodes embedded in a head band that can be worn by itself or within a regular or safety cap.	• Output displayed on a mobile phone or in cabin device using a fatigue speedometer with 4 levels. • Auditory and visual alerts are provided to the driver and can be sent to a central dispatcher.	Laboratory: • Good at detecting severe sleepiness as measured by 4 consecutive misses or more in a minute on the Oxford Sleepiness Resistance Test.[16] Field: • Smart cap signal acquired in field reliably represents EEG and varies as expected in association with circadian time of day patterns.[17]

This is not an exhaustive list of different drowsiness detection devices. Only those with a publicly available description and laboratory or field evidence are presented.

its lane (eg, lane centering). As these higher levels of automation are combined, the role and responsibilities of the driver start to change.

The Society for Automotive Engineers describes a taxonomy of the roles of the driver and the system as the technology becomes more sophisticated.[31] Critically, at lower levels (ie, Levels 1 and 2), although the driver might not be controlling the movements of the vehicle, the driver needs to remain engaged, vigilant, and take over control of the vehicle whenever necessary. Unfortunately, with the reduction in workload and passive monitoring of the driving environment, drivers are susceptible to lapses in vigilance. Hence, these systems might inadvertently contribute to instances of driver drowsiness and, by extension, decreased readiness to takeover when necessary.[32–34] More research is needed to understand the best strategies to keep drivers engaged while interacting with these systems.

At higher levels of automation (eg, Level 3), the driver might not need to actively monitor the traffic environment while the system is engaged. However, the driver must be ready to resume control of the vehicle when given notification. For such systems, the vehicle will need to provide ample warning for drivers who may be distracted, drowsy, or even asleep, in order for them to reacquaint themselves with the traffic context and safely resume control.

ROAD ADAPTATIONS

Delay or failure to take corrective measures, such as braking or steering maneuvers, increases the risk of crashes occurring at high speed, head-on collision, or the vehicle hitting a fixed obstacle, such as a tree. These behavioral and crash features are evident in sleepiness-related crashes due to a range of etiologies, including sleep apnea and shift workers,[6,35–37] with consequent higher rates of death and serious injury.[36,38,39] In some studies, almost 80% of sleepiness-related crashes are run off the road crashes, with absent or delayed steering correction.[36,40] In a recent Swedish study, almost 50% of all fatal road crashes were due to run off the road incidents, increasing to more than 60% for single-vehicle fatalities.[41] Given this high prevalence, road adaptations that prevent run off the road crashes or mitigate the crash impact and hence risk of death or injury are likely to be particularly beneficial for sleepiness-related crashes.

Road Adaptations for Run Off the Road Crashes

Several road adaptations successfully reduce the risk of a vehicle leaving the lane and having a run off the road crash. Audio-tactile lane markings, or rumble strips, mark the edge of lanes with an intermittent raised marker that results in vehicle vibration and noise when hit by tires. In a driving simulation study in shift workers, physiologic signs of sleepiness and impaired driving performance escalated before hitting the rumble strip.[42] There was an alerting effect evident after hitting the strip, with similar improvements in driving performance evident in field studies.[43] Importantly, however, the alerting effect was brief, lasting only 5 minutes. Interestingly, another study found there was a reduced time interval before rumble strips were hit on subsequent occasions and the alerting effect of hitting the strips dissipated.[44] This has raised concerns that rumble strips should not be considered a "cure" for sleepiness while driving, but act as a warning to institute countermeasures for sleepiness such as napping or caffeine.

Rumble strips reduce crash risk in real-world settings. The addition of rumble strips to center lines on undivided roads reduced overall crash risk by 14% and the risk of head-on or side swipe crashes (the main target of the intervention) by 25%.[45] The combination of both edgeline and centerline rumble strips produces greater reduction in crashes compared with either alone,[46] with overall crash reductions as great as 58% when they are combined with wide shoulders on the road.[47,48] They also specifically reduce run off the road crashes that are more likely to be due to sleepiness.[49] Rumble strips do not reduce crash severity, whereas other road adaptations such as barriers can impact severity of injuries.[50]

Barriers

Severe injury crashes on rural roads are dominated by road departures at high speed, with sleepiness-related crashes a key cause. It is also difficult to provide an adequate clear zone adjacent to highways in order to prevent collision with stationary objects or head-on collisions that dramatically increase the risk of severe injury and fatality. Roadside barriers can substantially reduce this risk, with different properties depending on the type of barrier, usually named rigid, semi-rigid, and flexible (**Fig. 2**).

Roadside barriers can reduce injury severity by deflecting or dissipating the energy of the vehicle and avoiding direct collisions with stationary objects or vehicles traveling in the opposite direction. Rigid, reinforced concrete barriers have the lowest rate of failure when hit, particularly for heavy vehicles, but result in the greatest impact and injury rate and more roll over incidents compared with other semi-rigid and flexible barriers.[51,52] For these reasons, it is preferable to target their

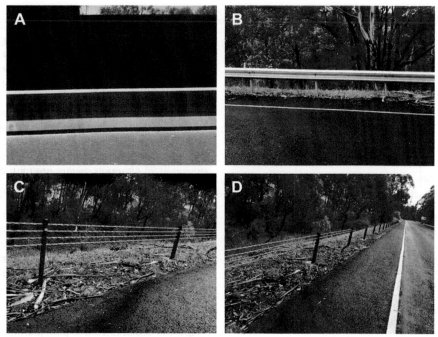

Fig. 2. Barrier types. (*A*) Concrete rigid barrier. (*B*) Semi-rigid barrier. (*C*) Flexible wire rope barrier. (*D*) Flexible barrier with wide shoulder on road.

installation for road sections where it is critical to avoid barrier failure, such as bridges. Installation of continuous flexible barriers consistently result in the greatest reductions in injury severity and fatalities from run off the road and head-on crashes. They are constructed of 3 or 4 wire ropes supported by weak posts from which they separate during a collision, resulting in the greatest dissipation of kinetic energy and vehicle re-direction.[52] Reductions in run off the road severe injury and fatal crashes as high as 83% have been reported on rural roads and highways fitted with flexible barriers.[51,53] In a large Swedish project, run off the road serious injury crashes and fatalities were reduced by 55% to 66% on highways fitted with wire rope flexible barriers[53] compared with a 36% reduction for roads with painted lines over the same time period. An Australian study found an 83% reduction in fatal and serious injury crashes on roads where flexible wire rope barriers were added (**Fig. 3**).[51] Total reported run off the road crashes reduced by 64% on the same roads, which is likely due at least in part to a range of other road safety measures introduced during the analysis period of 20 years. Nevertheless, there was a greater reduction in severe injury crashes, which was not evident for rigid and semi-rigid barriers (see **Fig. 3**).[51] Analysis of barrier crash data from high-speed roads suggests that injury severity for flexible barriers is approximately

half that from crashes where a stationary object is hit and substantially less than rigid and semi-rigid barriers or run off the road crashes when no object is hit.[54] Semi-rigid barriers also reduce injury severity compared with run off the road crashes where an object is hit.

Although the available crash data reflect overall reductions in run off the road and head-on crashes, a large proportion of these are likely to be related to sleepiness. Anecdotally, incidents have been reported in which flexible barriers have prevented almost certain fatalities after the driver has fallen asleep (**Fig. 4**).[55,56] As mentioned previously, wire rope flexible barriers are not effective at containing heavy vehicles traveling at speed. There have also been concerns regarding their safety for motorcyclists, given cases of injury if they hit the posts on the barriers. However, crash data analysis suggests that there is still an overall reduction in severe injury crashes for motorcyclists.[53]

ROAD ADAPTATIONS AND INFRASTRUCTURE TO ENHANCE ALERTNESS

Although run off the road crashes are a particularly relevant target for sleepiness-related driving impairment, variation in speed control, slow braking reaction times, or failure to brake and impaired visual attention may all contribute to

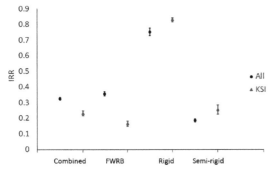

Fig. 3. Change in run off road crashes after road safety barrier installation incident rate ratio (IRR, and 95% confidence intervals) for all run off the road crashes (All) and killed or serious injury crashes (KSI) before and after road safety barrier installation in Western Australia over a 20-year period for all barrier types (Combined), flexible wire rope barriers (FWRB), and rigid and semi-rigid barriers. (*Data from* Chow K, Meuleners L. An evaluation of the effectiveness of flexible and non-flexible road safety barriers in Western Australia. Perth, Australia: Curtin-Monash Accident Research Centre;2016.)

safety critical events.[4,57] Several road infrastructure safety features may help alert sleepy drivers and reduce critical incidents arising from these abnormal behaviors. In a driving simulator study, drowsiness was induced by driving either after night shift or in older drivers during the afternoon circadian dip, resulting in greater variation in lateral lane position and percentage of time with eyes closed (PERCLOS).[58] Three interventions (transverse [in-lane] rumble strips, chevron line markings beside the road, and variable message signs about driver sleepiness) provided some improvements in PERCLOS and lateral lane position; however, these benefits were brief. Using transverse rumble strips proximally to critical locations appears to alert drivers to slow their speed.[59] An analysis of 15,000 speed observations at 12 sites found that transverse rumble strips reduced vehicle speeds by 9 to 12 kph when approaching pedestrian crosswalks on rural roads.[59] Crash

data from 366 sites from the same study found a 25% reduction in crashes. Simulated analysis of rural intersection crashes also suggests that combining transverse rumble strips with speed reduction on the approach to the intersection would provide the greatest reduction in injury severity.[60]

Breaks from driving, caffeine, and napping can help to reduce driver sleepiness; however, infrastructure needs to remind and enable drivers to use these strategies, particularly for long-distance driving.[61–63] Although drivers are usually aware of signs of sleepiness, they do not always predict impending episodes of microsleep.[64] Education regards indicators of sleepiness may assist drivers to decide when to use interventions for sleepiness and have been incorporated into roadside signage in some countries.[65,66] Appropriate roadside rest stops are required for breaks and napping, including rest room facilities and, for heavy vehicles in particular, adequate space to safely park vehicles and nap.[67] Providing access to rest stop maps can assist drivers to plan journeys.

SUMMARY

Sleepiness remains a major contributor to road crashes, with a higher rate of severe injury and death than most other causes. Although it is clearly important to optimize driver alertness, these strategies alone are unlikely to eliminate the problem. Vehicle and road safety adaptations are demonstrating great promise in reducing the frequency and severity of crashes, complementing work to optimize driver alertness. The physiologic changes that occur with increasing sleepiness and related changes in driver and vehicle behavior offer targets for these countermeasures. Driver sleepiness monitoring systems and vehicle adaptations, such as LDWs can capitalize on these features to provide alerts to drivers to use countermeasures for sleepiness. In cases of higher vehicle automation, these adaptations

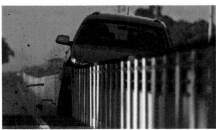
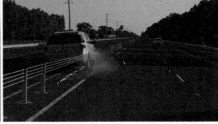

Fig. 4. Reconstruction of real-life run off the road incidents where severe collisions have been prevented by FWRB. (*Courtesy of* the Transport Accident Commission, Melbourne, Australia. https://www.towardszero.vic.gov.au/campaign/safety-barriers-save-lives; with permission.)

include actively taking over control of the vehicle to prevent run off the road incidents and institute emergency braking when the driver has failed to react. New technology, especially those offering partial or high automation, might lead to unintended consequences and the impact on drivers needs to be better understood, including ensuring the driver is fit to resume control of the vehicle as needed.

Similarly, roadway adaptation can offer warnings to drivers (eg, rumble strips) or can help mitigate the severity of crashes (barriers), with substantial proven benefits for run off the road crashes, many of which will be sleepiness related. Other infrastructure considerations also are important, such as encouraging drivers to use countermeasures through appropriate road signage and providing rest stops for breaks and sleep. The effectiveness of these adaptations varies for different road users. For example, flexible barriers that are highly effective in reducing injuries for standard vehicles are not effective for heavy vehicles. Although there is a substantial upfront cost for these road adaptations, there is growing evidence of long-term cost benefit when the reduced crash rate is taken into account.[47] In summary, vehicle and road adaptations offer great potential to help avoid or mitigate traffic crashes, including those due to driver sleepiness. Importantly, vehicle-based solutions to the drowsy driving problem should not be considered a panacea; other preventive countermeasures that address the problem at its source (ie, obtaining sufficient sleep) remain paramount.

REFERENCES

1. World Health Organization UNRSC. Global plan for the decade of action for road safety 2011–2020. Geneva (Switzerland): World Health Organisation; 2011. Availble at: www.who.int/roadsafety/decade_of_action/.
2. Stigson H, Hill J. Use of car crashes resulting in fatal and serious injuries to analyze a safe road transport system model and to identify system weaknesses. Traffic Inj Prev 2009;10(5):441–50.
3. Stigson H, Krafft M, Tingvall C. Use of fatal real-life crashes to analyze a safe road transport system model, including the road user, the vehicle, and the road. Traffic Inj Prev 2008;9(5):463–71.
4. Shiferaw BA, Downey LA, Westlake J, et al. Stationary gaze entropy predicts lane departure events in sleep-deprived drivers. Sci Rep 2018;8(1):2220.
5. Sandberg D, Anund A, Fors C, et al. The characteristics of sleepiness during real driving at night–a study of driving performance, physiology and subjective experience. Sleep 2011;34(10):1317–25.
6. Lee ML, Howard ME, Horrey WJ, et al. High risk of near-crash driving events following night-shift work. Proc Natl Acad Sci U S A 2016;113(1):176–81.
7. Hallvig D, Anund A, Fors C, et al. Real driving at night - predicting lane departures from physiological and subjective sleepiness. Biol Psychol 2014;101: 18–23.
8. Liang Y, Horrey WJ, Howard ME, et al. Prediction of drowsiness events in night shift workers during morning driving. Accid Anal Prev 2019;126:105–14.
9. Ftouni S, Sletten TL, Howard M, et al. Objective and subjective measures of sleepiness, and their associations with on-road driving events in shift workers. J Sleep Res 2013;22(1):58–69.
10. Dawson D, Searle AK, Paterson JL. Look before you (s)leep: evaluating the use of fatigue detection technologies within a fatigue risk management system for the road transport industry. Sleep Med Rev 2014;18(2):141–52.
11. Aidman E, Chadunow C, Johnson K, et al. Real-time driver drowsiness feedback improves driver alertness and self-reported driving performance. Accid Anal Prev 2015;81:8–13.
12. Fitzharris M, Liu S, Stephens AN, et al. The relative importance of real-time in-cab and external feedback in managing fatigue in real-world commercial transport operations. Traffic Inj Prev 2017;18:S71–8.
13. Lal SKL, Craig A. A critical review of the psychophysiology of driver fatigue. Biol Psychol 2001;55: 173–94.
14. Phipps-Nelson JO, Redman JR, Rajaratnam SMW. Temporal profile of prolonged, night-time driving performance: breaks from driving temporarily reduce time-on-task fatigue but not sleepiness. J Sleep Res 2011;20:404–15.
15. Perrier J, Jongen S, Vuurman E, et al. Driving performance and EEG fluctuations during on-the-road driving following sleep deprivation. Biol Psychol 2016;121:1–11.
16. Rajaratnam SMW, Howard ME. Evaluation of the SmartCap technology to monitor drowsiness in healthy volunteers exposed to sleep restriction – Relationship between the SmartCap fatigue algorithm and frequent misses on the Osler Test. Clayton: Monash University; 2011. Available at: http://www.smartcaptech.com/wp-content/uploads/Monash-Fatigue-Assessment-full.pdf.
17. Opazo Fuenzalida CA, Holgado San Martín A. Evaluation of "SmartCap" tecnology designed to monitor on-line the fatigue level of workers. Santiago, (Chile): School of Medicine, University of Chile; 2015.
18. Jackson ML, Kennedy GA, Clarke C, et al. The utility of automated measures of ocular metrics for detecting driver drowsiness during extended wakefulness. Accid Anal Prev 2016;87:127–33.
19. Fairclough SH, Graham R. Impairment of driving performance caused by sleep deprivation or

alcohol: a comparative study. Hum Factors 1999; 41(1):118–28.

20. Friedrichs F, Yang B. Drowsiness monitoring by steering and lane data based features under real driving conditions 18th European Signal Processing Conference. Aalborg, (Denmark): IEEE; 2010.

21. Group FMI. ASTiD summary of operation. 2018. Available at: https://fmiltd.co.uk/astid.html. Accessed January 14, 2019.

22. Dinges D, Maislin G, Brewster R, et al. Pilot test of fatigue management technologies. Transport Research Record: Journal of the Transportation Research Board 2005;1922:175–82.

23. Yanagisawa M, Swanson E, Azeredo P, et al. Estimation of potential safety benefits for pedestrian crash avoidance/mitigation systems. Washington, D.C.: National Highway Traffic Safety Administration; 2017.

24. Jermakian JS. Crash avoidance potential of four passenger vehicle technologies. Accid Anal Prev 2011;43(3):732–40.

25. Cicchino JB. Effectiveness of forward collision warning and autonomous emergency braking systems in reducing front-to-rear crash rates. Accid Anal Prev 2017;99(Pt A):142–52.

26. Benson AJ, Tefft BC, Svancara AM, et al. Potential reductions in crashes, injuries, and deaths from large-scale deployment of advanced driver assistance systems. Washington, D.C: AAA Foundation for Traffic Safety; 2018.

27. Gaspar JG, Schwarz j-CW, Brown TL, et al. Gaze position modulates the effectiveness of forward collision warnings for drowsy drivers. Accid Anal Prev 2019;126:25–30.

28. Cicchino JB. Effects of lane departure warning on police-reported crash rates. J Safety Res 2018;66: 61–70.

29. Tefft BC. Prevalence of motor vehicle crashes involving drowsy drivers, United States, 1999–2008. Accid Anal Prev 2012;45:180–6.

30. Rimini-Doering M, Altmueller T, Ladstaetter U, et al. Effects of lane departure warning on drowsy drivers' performance and state in a simulator. Paper presented at: Third International Driving Symposium on Human Factors in Driver Assessment, Training and Vehicle Design. Iowa City, June 28, 2005.

31. SAE. Taxonomy and definitions for terms related to driving automation systems for on-road motor vehicles. Warrendale (PA): Society for Automotive Engineers; 2018.

32. Cunningham M, Regan MA. Autonomous vehicles: human factors issues and future research. Paper presented at: Australasian Road Safety Conference. Gold Coast, Australia, October 14, 2015.

33. Schömig N, Hargutt V, Neukum A, et al. The interaction between highly automated driving and the development of drowsiness. Procedia Manuf 2015; 3:6652–9.

34. de Winter JCF, Happee R, Martens MH, et al. Effects of adaptive cruise control and highly automated driving on workload and situation awareness: a review of the empirical evidence. Transport Res F Traffic Psychol Behav 2014;27: 196–217.

35. Mazza S, Pepin JL, Naegele B, et al. Driving ability in sleep apnoea patients before and after CPAP treatment: evaluation on a road safety platform. Eur Respir J 2006;28(5):1020–8.

36. Pack AI, Pack AM, Rodgman E, et al. Characteristics of crashes attributed to the driver having fallen asleep. Accid Anal Prev 1995;27(6): 769–75.

37. Chen Z, Wu C, Zhong M, et al. Identification of common features of vehicle motion under drowsy/distracted driving: a case study in Wuhan, China. Accid Anal Prev 2015;81:251–9.

38. Philip P, Vervialle F, Le Breton P, et al. Fatigue, alcohol, and serious road crashes in France: factorial study of national data. BMJ 2001;322(7290): 829–30.

39. Mulgrew AT, Nasvadi G, Butt A, et al. Risk and severity of motor vehicle crashes in patients with obstructive sleep apnoea/hypopnoea. Thorax 2008;63(6):536–41.

40. Woolley J, Stokes C, Turner B, et al. Towards safe system infrastructure. Sydney (Australia): Austro-ads; 2018.

41. Sternlund S. The safety potential of lane departure warning systems—a descriptive real-world study of fatal lane departure passenger car crashes in Sweden. Traffic Inj Prev 2017;18(sup1):S18–s23.

42. Anund A, Kecklund G, Vadeby A, et al. The alerting effect of hitting a rumble strip—a simulator study with sleepy drivers. Accid Anal Prev 2008;40(6):1970–6.

43. Rosey F, Auberlet JM, Bertrand J, et al. Impact of perceptual treatments on lateral control during driving on crest vertical curves: a driving simulator study. Accid Anal Prev 2008;40(4):1513–23.

44. Watling CN, Akerstedt T, Kecklund G, et al. Do repeated rumble strip hits improve driver alertness? J Sleep Res 2016;25(2):241–7.

45. Persaud BN, Retting RA, Lyon CA. Crash reduction following installation of centerline rumble strips on rural two-lane roads. Accid Anal Prev 2004;36(6): 1073–9.

46. Hatfield J, Murphy S, Job RF, et al. The effectiveness of audio-tactile lane-marking in reducing various types of crash: a review of evidence, template for evaluation, and preliminary findings from Australia. Accid Anal Prev 2009;41(3):365–79.

47. Meuleners LB, Hendrie D, Lee AH. Effectiveness of sealed shoulders and audible edge lines in Western Australia. Traffic Inj Prev 2011;12(2):201–5.

48. Park J, Abdel-Aty M, Lee C. Exploration and comparison of crash modification factors for multiple treatments on rural multilane roadways. Accid Anal Prev 2014;70:167–77.

49. Khan M, Abdel-Rahim A, Williams CJ. Potential crash reduction benefits of shoulder rumble strips in two-lane rural highways. Accid Anal Prev 2015;75:35–42.

50. Wu KF, Donnell ET, Aguero-Valverde J. Relating crash frequency and severity: evaluating the effectiveness of shoulder rumble strips on reducing fatal and major injury crashes. Accid Anal Prev 2014;67: 86–95.

51. Chow K, Meuleners L. An evaluation of the effectiveness of flexible and non-flexible road safety barriers in Western Australia. Perth (Australia): Curtin-Monash Accident Research Centre; 2016.

52. Hammonds B, Troutbeck R. Crash test outcomes for three generic barrier types. 25th ARRB Conference. Perth, Australia, September 23, 2012.

53. Carlsson A. Evaluation of 2+1 roads with cable barriers: final report 2009. p. 1–28. Available at: https://www.diva-portal.org/smash/get/diva2:670552/ FULLTEXT01.pdf. Accessed January 14, 2019.

54. Jurewicz C, Steinmetz L. Crash performance of safety barriers on high-speed roads. J Australas Coll Road Saf 2012;23(3):37–44.

55. TAC. Saving lives – Melba Highway wire rope barrier. 2016. Available at: http://www.tac.vic.gov.au/about-the-tac/media-room/news-and-events/2016/saving-lives-melba-highway-wire-rope-barrier. Accessed January 31, 2019.

56. TAC. Safety barriers save lives. 2018. Available at: https://www.facebook.com/TransportAccident Commission/. Accessed January 31, 2019.

57. Dingus T, Klauer S, Neale V, et al. The 100-car naturalistic driving study. Springfield (VA): Virginia Tech Transportation Institute, NHTSA; 2006. DOT HS 810593.

58. Merat N, Jamson AH. The effect of three low-cost engineering treatments on driver fatigue: a driving simulator study. Accid Anal Prev 2013; 50:8–15.

59. Liu P, Huang J, Wang W, et al. Effects of transverse rumble strips on safety of pedestrian crosswalks on rural roads in China. Accid Anal Prev 2011;43(6): 1947–54.

60. Peiris S, Corben B, Nieuwesteeg M, et al. Evaluation of alternative intersection treatments at rural crossroads using simulation software. Traffic Inj Prev 2018;19(sup2):S1–7.

61. Horne JA, Reyner LA. Counteracting driver sleepiness: effects of napping, caffeine, and placebo. Psychophysiology 1996;33(3):306–9.

62. Sharwood LN, Elkington J, Meuleners L, et al. Use of caffeinated substances and risk of crashes in long distance drivers of commercial vehicles: case-control study. BMJ 2013;346:f1140.

63. Chen C, Xie Y. The impacts of multiple rest-break periods on commercial truck driver's crash risk. J Safety Res 2014;48:87–93.

64. Kaplan KA, Itoi A, Dement WC. Awareness of sleepiness and ability to predict sleep onset: can drivers avoid falling asleep at the wheel? Sleep Med 2007;9(1):71–9.

65. Alvaro PK, Burnett NM, Kennedy GA, et al. Driver education: enhancing knowledge of sleep, fatigue and risky behaviour to improve decision making in young drivers. Accid Anal Prev 2018; 112:77–83.

66. Howard ME, Jackson ML, Berlowitz D, et al. Specific sleepiness symptoms are indicators of performance impairment during sleep deprivation. Accid Anal Prev 2014;62:1–8.

67. Munala G, Maina K. Rest stops as a planning engineering option to fatigue. JAGST 2012;14(1): 204–18.

68. Anderson C, Chang AM, Sullivan JP, et al. Assessment of drowsiness based on ocular parameters detected by infrared reflectance oculography. J Clin Sleep Med 2013;9(9):907–20.

69. Wilkinson VE, Jackson ML, Westlake J, et al. The accuracy of eyelid movement parameters for drowsiness detection. J Clin Sleep Med 2013;9(12): 1315–24.

70. Caterpillar Inc. Operator Fatigue: Detection Technology Review. Available at. https://www.slideshare. net/willred/cat-fatigue-technology-report-2008.

Sleepiness and Driving
The Role of Official Regulation

Walter T. McNicholas, MD[a,b,*]

KEYWORDS

- Sleepiness • Driving regulations • Motor vehicle accidents • Obstructive sleep apnea

KEY POINTS

- Sleepiness is a major contributing factor in approximately 20% of highway accidents, which justifies official measures to regulate drivers with this presentation.
- The most common medical cause of excessive sleepiness is obstructive sleep apnea (OSA), which confers an approximate 3-fold increased risk of driving accident, yet effective therapy largely removes this risk.
- Several jurisdictions, notably the European Union and Australia, have implemented official measures to regulate driving in patients with OSA, which prohibit driving in patients with moderate OSA or severe OSA associated with sleepiness but permit driving once the disorder is effectively treated.
- Education of all relevant stakeholders is an important component of effective regulation, including educating affected patients on the benefits of diagnosis and treatment, employers in the trucking industry on the benefits of screening, and the police on the reporting of motor vehicle accidents where sleepiness is a contributing factor.

INTRODUCTION

There are specific characteristics pertaining to the driver that increase the likelihood of having a motor vehicle accident (MVA), which include excessive speed and alcohol consumption, and every developed country has specific regulations limiting highway speed and alcohol level while driving. Sleep disturbances and disorders also represent a major risk factor for MVA, and recognition of this risk has grown progressively over recent decades.[1] The scale of the problem is demonstrated by reports, indicating that approximately 20% of serious MVAs have driver fatigue or sleepiness as a major contributing factor.[2–4] Furthermore, a recent European survey of 12,434 drivers reported that the average prevalence of falling asleep at the wheel in the previous 2 years was 17% and 7% of those falling asleep experienced a sleep-related accident.[5] The growing recognition of the risk of drowsy driving has led regulatory authorities in some countries to implement restrictions on driver licensing for patients with specific sleep-related disorders, such as obstructive sleep apnea (OSA), notably the regulations recently introduced by the European Union (EU) on driving in OSA.[6] This development is particularly important as the increased MVA risk associated with OSA exceeds the risk associated with many other medical disorders already specified in the driving license regulations of many jurisdictions.[7] General restrictions targeting sleepy drivers, however, are difficult to formulate because it is difficult to reliably quantify sleepiness in contrast to the highly specific criteria available for speed and alcohol levels.

Conflict of Interest: None.
[a] Department of Respiratory and Sleep Medicine, School of Medicine, University College Dublin, St. Vincent's Hospital Group, Elm Park, Dublin 4, Ireland; [b] First Affiliated Hospital of Guangzhou Medical University, Guangzhou, China
* Department of Respiratory and Sleep Medicine, St. Vincent's Hospital, Elm Park, Dublin 4, Ireland.
E-mail address: walter.mcnicholas@ucd.ie

Sleep Med Clin 14 (2019) 491–498
https://doi.org/10.1016/j.jsmc.2019.08.006

PUBLIC HEALTH AND SAFETY

The increased risk of MVA in sleepy drivers has important implications for the safety of both the driver and others in the vehicle and also for the general public traveling on highways, especially because MVAs occurring because of sleepiness are more likely to result in more severe collisions with a higher likelihood of serious injury or death due to absent or poor avoidance measures by the driver who falls asleep at the wheel.[3,8,9] Further factors contributing to the likelihood of a major collision include that MVAs as a result of sleepiness are more likely on major highways and to involve long-haul truck drivers.[10–12] Thus, the public safety implications of sleepy driving place an onus on regulatory authorities to protect the general public and to take appropriate measures to restrict the ability of drivers susceptible to sleepiness from continuing to drive unless and until the underlying disorder is adequately treated.

One limitation in an MVA relating to sleepiness is the frequent lack of information on the characteristics of the accident scene that might indicate sleepiness as a causal factor in the accident.[13] Relating a crash to drowsy driving relies almost entirely on police crash reports and associated hospital records. In many jurisdictions, however, sleepiness is not identified as a source of accidents in the police report and many police officers are unaware of disorders predisposing to MVA, such as OSA. Thus, sleepiness as a factor in MVAs is likely under-reported and education of policing authorities on the possibility of sleepiness-induced MVA is necessary to obtain accurate statistics. Relevant factors indicating sleepiness as a likely factor in an MVA involving a sleepy driver include absence of brake marks, a single-vehicle accident, rear-end or head-on collision, MVA during the height of sleepiness hours (midafternoon and night hours), and MVA resulting in injuries or fatalities.

RESPONSIBILITIES OF THE TREATING PHYSICIAN AND AFFECTED PATIENT

Where an underlying medical disorder, such as OSA or narcolepsy, is responsible for sleepiness, the respective responsibilities of the affected patient and the treating physician represent an important consideration and have been the subject of discussion over many years. Although the treating physician has a responsibility to warn the patient suffering excessive daytime sleepiness (EDS) of the risk of MVA while driving and to advise against driving if EDS is deemed sufficient to increase driving risk, there is an understandable reluctance among physicians to have a legal responsibility placed on them to inform regulatory authorities or to be legally responsible in the event of an MVA caused by their patient due to sleepiness. Sleepy drivers must take responsibility for their own actions and avoid driving while sleepy. Many drivers have limited appreciation, however, of their level of sleepiness and its consequences, which is well demonstrated by reports that many drivers having an MVA due to sleepiness give a history of several near-miss events beforehand[14] and near-miss events due to sleepiness more likely associated with OSA than with acute sleep deprivation.[15]

SLEEP DISTURBANCES AND DISORDERS ASSOCIATED WITH SLEEPINESS AND DRIVING RISK

Sleep disturbances and disorder with sleepiness include poor lifestyle, inadequate sleep time, and various medical disorders that are associated with EDS, including OSA, narcolepsy, and periodic leg movement disorder. The increased risk of MVA in patients with narcolepsy is at least twice the general population of drivers and the risk is reduced only with long-term therapy for the disorder.[16] Modafinil therapy has been demonstrated to improve real driving performance in patients with narcolepsy.[17]

Lifestyle factors include time of day (afternoon and night-time driving), shift work, sedative medications, poor sleep hygiene, and alcohol use. Modern society often is associated with sleep restriction, and a recent report from the US Centers for Disease Control and Prevention indicated that 11.8% of 444,306 respondents to a random survey of the adult US population indicated an average of less than or equal to 5 hours sleep.[18] Sleep deficiency due to inadequate sleep time or to medical disorders, such as OSA, has been strongly associated with increased MVA rate in the general population.[19,20] A report from France comparing sleep patterns and sleepiness among drivers between 1996 and 2011 indicated that drivers surveyed in 2011 reported shorter sleep duration and higher levels of sleepiness compared with in 1996, and drivers in 2011 reported a 2.5 times greater rate of the Epworth Sleepiness Scale (ESS) score greater than 15, indicating severe sleepiness.[21] Young drivers seem especially prone to MVA because of sleep deficit[22] whereas older drivers do not seem to be at increased risk.[23] Excessive sleep duration also seems to represent a risk factor for MVA.[2]

The most prevalent medical disorder associated with increased accident risk is OSA, which affects up to 10% of the adult population[24] and is more than 100 times more prevalent than narcolepsy, which also represents a major accident risk.[25] Thus, it should not be surprising that most interest in the topic of medical disorders associated with sleepiness and driving risk has focused on OSA. Although not universally accepted, the balance of evidence favors the level of EDS as the most important parameter of OSA severity that determines MVA risk.[26–28] The importance of recognizing medical disorders associated with EDS is underlined by the efficacy of treatment, especially continuous positive airway pressure (CPAP) therapy in patients with OSA, which is most effective in symptom control.[29] There are many published reports indicating that the increased risk of MVA associated with OSA is reduced to general population levels with effective therapy,[28,30–32] which provides a clear basis for regulatory measures to identify and require adequate treatment of OSA in affected drivers. The beneficial impact of CPAP therapy on driving risk in a cluster analysis of OSA seems largely restricted to the excessive sleepiness phenotype.[33] The increased accident risk in drivers with OSA may be compounded by lifestyle factors, and the report of Garbarino and coauthors[34] indicates that sleep restriction greatly increases the MVA risk in commercial drivers suffering from OSA. In another report, these investigators demonstrated that insomnia is highly prevalent in truck drivers and is associated with a higher rate of MVA.[35] Alcohol consumption substantially increases the MVA risk in drivers with OSA.[36,37]

REGULATION OF FITNESS TO DRIVE IN DISORDERS ASSOCIATED WITH SLEEPINESS

Several diseases are associated with an increased prevalence of MVA compared with the general population, including diabetes mellitus, cardiovascular diseases, cerebrovascular diseases, psychiatric conditions, and uncorrected visual defects.[38] Based on these associations, licensing authorities in many countries have restricted the right to drive in individuals suffering from these established causes of increased accident risk. Each country has developed its own list of diseases in this context. Drivers typically are required to declare if they suffer from a listed disease and may need to demonstrate that corrective measures have been undertaken or that the disease does not adversely affect their ability to drive before an unrestricted driving license is issued. Authorities may limit the duration or extension of the license concerned.

Regulations to restrict the ability to drive of individuals with medical disorders or other factors associated with sleepiness are limited by the difficulty in establishing reliable criteria to assess and quantify this variable. The most commonly used measure is subjective using questionnaires, such as the ESS score.[39] Any subjective measure is open to reporting bias, however, which is especially likely in professional drivers who rely on a valid driving license for continuing employment. Furthermore, the ESS may not be the most reliable measure of sleepiness while driving because the score assesses sleepiness in passive situations, whereas sleepiness at the wheel applies to a highly active setting of driving a vehicle and requiring a high level of concentration.[1] This aspect may account for inconsistent findings in previous reports regarding the relationship between ESS score and accident risk and supports additional questioning regarding sleepiness at the wheel in this assessment. Objective measures, such as multiple sleep latency testing and maintenance of wakefulness testing, are more reliable but are time consuming and labor intensive.[26] An alternative is the driving simulator, which evaluates driver attention and reaction time where sleepiness is only one variable that may contribute to poor performance and has limited correlation with on road performance in sleepy drivers,[40] although treatment of OSA patients with CPAP has been associated with improved driving simulator performance.[30]

Obstructive Sleep Apnea

Some jurisdictions have implemented regulations to limit the ability of OSA patients to drive unless the disorder is effectively treated. The regulations concerned should not be based only on the objective severity of OSA in a sleep test, because the increased risk of MVA associated with OSA relates most closely to the associated level of sleepiness.[34] This aspect is important because there is a poor association between OSA severity measured by the apnea-hypopnea frequency per hour (apnea-hypopnea index [AHI]) in a sleep test and the subjective level of sleepiness reported by measures, such as the ESS.[41,42] Thus, regulations should include both AHI and level of sleepiness, especially while driving. Furthermore, the medical assessment of fitness to drive in patients with OSA should be made by a clinician with competence and experience in treating such patients. The ultimate responsibility for determining fitness to drive a vehicle (including a conditional license) depends on the relevant administrative authority with decisions supported by medical reports and recommendations of specialized physicians or structures.[43] Individual patients should receive verbal and/or written information on their condition and its potential impact on fitness to drive and they should be advised to report such information to the relevant authority responsible for driving license delivery.

A special consideration is the occupational driver, where the employer has a role in ensuring competent and safe drivers.[44] The potential benefits of employers playing an active role in promoting OSA diagnosis and treatment are well demonstrated by the report of Burks and coauthors,[45] who analyzed data from an employer-mandated program to screen, diagnose, and monitor OSA treatment adherence in the US trucking industry. OSA-positive drivers who did not accept CPAP therapy had an MVA rate 5-fold greater than matched controls, whereas the MVA rate of OSA drivers fully compliant with CPAP therapy was no different to controls. Furthermore, a majority of nonadherent CPAP-treated OSA patients subsequently left employment in the trucking industry, suggesting that the program had the added advantage of weeding out patients with significant OSA who represent a driving risk. Although the same criteria of OSA severity can apply to commercial and private drivers, commercial drivers warrant closer monitoring of treatment compliance and efficacy, especially long-haul truck drivers, because they pose a greater potential risk on public highways relating to distances driven and the size of the vehicle involved.

An important development in the context of regulating driver licensing in OSA was the establishment in 2012 of a working group by the Transport and Mobility Directorate of the European Commission to examine the driving risk of patients with OSA and to advise the Commission on appropriate regulations that could be implemented throughout the EU in this context. This initiative was the culmination of many years' representation to the Commission by leading experts on sleep disorders and driving safety.[46] The working group issued a report in 2013,[43] which led to an official EU directive in 2014 that became mandatory for implementation by all EU member states in January 2016, and thus applies to a population over 500 million.[6,47] The directive states as follows:

1. In the following paragraphs, a moderate OSA syndrome corresponds to a number of apneas and hypopneas per hour (AHI) between 15 and 29 and a severe OSA syndrome corresponds to an AHI of 30 or more, both associated with EDS.
2. Applicants or drivers in whom a moderate or severe OSA syndrome is suspected shall be referred to further authorized medical advice before a driving license is issued or renewed. They may be advised not to drive until confirmation of the diagnosis.
3. Driving licenses may be issued to applicants or drivers with moderate or severe OSA syndrome who show adequate control of their condition and compliance with appropriate treatment and improvement of sleepiness, if any, confirmed by authorized medical opinion.
4. Applicants or drivers with moderate or severe OSA syndrome under treatment shall be subject to a periodic medical review, at intervals not exceeding 3 years for drivers of group 1 and 1 year for drivers of group 2, with a view to establishing the level of compliance with the treatment, the need for continuing the treatment, and continued good vigilance.

The overarching objective of this directive is to prevent patients with untreated OSA who report sleepiness while driving from continuing to drive until the disorder is effectively treated. The directive does not specify the level of sleepiness that should apply in OSA, although some EU member states have qualified sleepiness in their national regulations as sleepiness while driving. The directive can be viewed as a minimum standard because either sleepiness or high AHI alone is not enough to preclude driving.

In most other jurisdictions, the regulatory provisions regarding driver licensing in disorders associated with EDS such as OSA are less well developed. In the United States, federal regulations introduced in 2016 by the Federal Motor Carrier Safety Administration regarding moderate OSA and severe OSA among individuals in safety-sensitive positions in highway transportation were subsequently rescinded in 2017. Individual states, however, have implemented varying levels of regulation for drowsy driving, and Arkansas and New Jersey have laws that make sleep-deprived driving a criminal offense.[48] Other states implement awareness campaigns to limit drowsy driving but do not have official regulations. Canada has no official regulation regarding driving and OSA. Japan also has no official regulations regarding drowsy driving or OSA although has supported awareness initiatives on the risk of OSA and sleepiness as a driving risk.

Australia has implemented specific regulations regarding driving in subjects with sleepiness that also refer to OSA.[49] These regulations specify that a person is not fit to hold an unconditional license if (1) the person has OSA (on a diagnostic sleep study and moderate to severe EDS), (2) the person has frequent self-reported episodes of sleepiness or drowsiness while driving or the person has had 1 or more motor vehicle crashes caused by inattention or sleepiness, or (4) the person, in opinion of the treating doctor, represents a significant driving risk as a result of a sleep disorder. A conditional license may be considered by the driver licensing authority subject to periodic review, considering the nature of the driving task and information provided by the treating doctor as to whether the following criteria are met: the person is compliant with treatment and the response to treatment is satisfactory.

These Australian regulations are broader than the European regulations because they also refer to sleepiness while driving separately from OSA.

Other Disorders Associated with Sleepiness

Although narcolepsy is substantially less prevalent than OSA, the major MVA risk associated with this disorder[25,50] has led several jurisdictions to prohibit drivers with this disorder from driving until the manifestations have been effectively treated. In contrast to OSA, these regulations typically require that relevant symptoms of EDS and cataplexy be satisfactorily controlled for a defined period of 3 months to 6 months and physician certification of adequate treatment is required.

Excessive sleepiness in the absence of a defined medical disorder is hard to regulate because of the difficulty in establishing objective criteria for EDS, although the Australian regulations include reference to sleepiness alone. Some jurisdictions, however, make it a criminal offense if a driver is the cause of a major MVA resulting in death or injury where EDS is proved the major contributing factor.[48]

EFFECTIVE IMPLEMENTATION OF REGULATIONS AND ROLE OF EDUCATION

There is understandable concern that many drivers may not admit to significant sleepiness because of the risk of losing their license, which may apply particularly to commercial drivers who risk losing their livelihood if the driving license is withdrawn. Thus, subjective sleepiness questionnaires, such as the ESS, have significant limitations of potential reporting bias. This aspect also raises concern that the directive could inhibit drivers from seeking diagnosis and treatment of the disorder and thus be counterproductive. Thus, appropriate measures to educate and reassure potential OSA sufferers and treating clinicians on the benefits of diagnosis and treatment become a priority in the effective implementation of these regulations.

The EU directive takes a carrot-and-stick approach to regulation by not only banning potentially dangerous drivers but also encouraging effective treatment by permitting immediate resumption of driving in treatment compliant OSA patients. The directive has led, however, to some confusion among patients with OSA and among many clinicians treating such patients.[51] Thus, education of patients and treating clinicians represents an important component of this regulatory process. An important goal in the implementation of regulations for drivers with OSA is to not discourage such patients from seeking diagnosis and treatment, which applies especially to OSA patients who are professional drivers. Thus, education should particularly stress the carrot of benefit to driving safety associated with effective treatment and not place excessive emphasis on the stick of a driving ban because this applies only to patients who are sleepy and do not comply with treatment. Furthermore, there is a strong case for education of employers in the transport industry in the value of diagnosis and treatment of patients with OSA because the evidence strongly supports such drivers being safer and more productive.[45] The role of screening drivers for disorders, such as OSA, by employers is a topical subject and increasingly regarded as a worthwhile objective.[45,52–54] Screening programs and related policies should ensure, however, that appropriate measures of driving risk should be identified, especially the level of sleepiness, and not simply based on syndrome severity determined by the AHI. Additional assessments, such as psychomotor vigilance testing, may provide useful additional information on sleepiness and impaired vigilance, which may be appropriate in selected populations.[55]

A recent report by Grote and coauthors[56] provides further interesting and potentially important information on the certification of fitness to drive in OSA patients. The investigators reported that OSA patients treated with CPAP undergoing certification to drive had higher CPAP compliance and greater reduction in ESS score than a control group of similarly treated OSA patients already in possession of a valid driving license.[56] These data suggest that the requirement for certification provides a motivation to be more compliant with therapy with associated greater improvement in symptom control and thus safer driving.[57]

THE FUTURE

Current practice relating to driver assessment in disorders associated with sleepiness is compromised by the lack of reliable and easily implemented tools for the evaluation of sleepiness. There is an urgent requirement for objective tools to assess driving impairment due to EDS that can be applied to large groups of drivers, especially in the transport industry. Furthermore, the relative contribution of AHI and EDS to MVA risk in OSA patients is not fully clear.

The future direction of regulations for driver licensing in patients who experience EDS due to medical disorders, such as OSA, or lifestyle factors, such as inadequate sleep, is likely to be influenced by technological developments in vehicles and highways that compensate for driver inattention and drowsiness. The ultimate compensation is autonomous vehicles, which currently are under development but are unlikely to be in widespread use for the foreseeable future. Thus, cooperation between experts in sleep disorders and those involved in vehicle development and highway safety should be encouraged to facilitate measures to optimize road safety. Efforts have begun in this area as demonstrated by a recent forum established by the US National Highway Traffic Safety Administration, which brought together motor vehicle and highway safety experts with sleep/circadian science experts and the sleep medicine community seeking to establish a partnership in which longstanding knowledge and experience could be combined to effectively address the challenge of eliminating drowsy driving.[13]

REFERENCES

1. Bioulac S, Franchi J-AM, Arnaud M, et al. Risk of motor vehicle accidents related to sleepiness at the wheel: a systematic review and meta-analysis. Sleep 2017;40(10):zsx134.
2. Maia Q, Grandner MA, Findley J, et al. Short and long sleep duration and risk of drowsy driving and the role of subjective sleep insufficiency. Accid Anal Prev 2013;59:618–22.
3. Czeisler CA, Wickwire EM, Barger LK, et al. Sleep-deprived motor vehicle operators are unfit to drive: a multidisciplinary expert consensus statement on drowsy driving. Sleep Health 2016;2(2):94–9.
4. Tefft BC. Prevalence of motor vehicle crashes involving drowsy drivers, United States, 1999–2008. Accid Anal Prev 2012;45:180–6.
5. Gonçalves M, Amici R, Lucas R, et al. Sleepiness at the wheel across Europe: a survey of 19 countries. J Sleep Res 2015;24(3):242–53.
6. Bonsignore MR, Randerath W, Riha R, et al. New rules on driver licensing for patients with obstructive sleep apnea: European Union Directive 2014/85/EU. J Sleep Res 2016;25(1):3–4.
7. Vaa T. Impairments, diseases, age and their relative risks of accident involvement: results from a meta-analysis. Oslo (Norway): Institute of Transport Economics; 2003.
8. Strohl KP, Brown DB, Collop N, et al. An official American Thoracic Society clinical practice guideline: sleep apnea, sleepiness, and driving risk in noncommercial drivers. An update of a 1994 statement. Am J Respir Crit Care Med 2013;187(11):1259–66.
9. Mulgrew AT, Nasvadi G, Butt A, et al. Risk and severity of motor vehicle crashes in patients with obstructive sleep apnoea/hypopnoea. Thorax 2008;63(6):536–41.
10. Meuleners L, Fraser ML, Govorko MH, et al. Obstructive sleep apnea, health-related factors, and long distance heavy vehicle crashes in Western Australia: a case control study. J Clin Sleep Med 2015;11(4):413–8.
11. Mitler MM, Miller JC, Lipsitz JJ, et al. The sleep of long-haul truck drivers. N Engl J Med 1997;337(11):755–62.
12. Pack AI, Maislin G, Staley B, et al. Impaired performance in commercial drivers. Am J Respir Crit Care Med 2006;174(4):446–54.
13. Higgins JS, Rosekind MR, Austin R, et al. Asleep at the wheel—the road to addressing drowsy driving. Sleep 2017;40(2).
14. Watson NF, Morgenthaler T, Chervin R, et al. Confronting drowsy driving: the american academy of sleep medicine perspective. J Clin Sleep Med 2015;11(11):1335–6.
15. Quera Salva MA, Barbot F, Hartley S, et al. Sleep disorders, sleepiness, and near-miss accidents among long-distance highway drivers in the summertime. Sleep Med 2014;15(1):23–6.
16. Pizza F, Jaussent I, Lopez R, et al. Car crashes and central disorders of hypersomnolence: a French study. PLoS One 2015;10(6):e0129386.
17. Capelli A, Chaufton C, Philip P, et al. Modafinil improves real driving performance in patients with hypersomnia: a randomized double-blind placebo-controlled crossover clinical trial. Sleep 2014;37(3):483–7.
18. Liu YWA, Chapman DP, Cunningham TJ, et al. Prevalence of healthy sleep duration among adults–United States, 2014. MMWR Morb Mortal Wkly Rep 2016;65(6):137–41.
19. Gottlieb DJ, Ellenbogen JM, Bianchi MT, et al. Sleep deficiency and motor vehicle crash risk in the general population: a prospective cohort study. BMC Med 2018;16:44.
20. Philip P, Chaufton C, Orriols L, et al. Complaints of poor sleep and risk of traffic accidents: a population-based case-control study. PLoS One 2014;9(12):e114102.
21. Quera-Salva MA, Hartley S, Sauvagnac-Quera R, et al. Association between reported sleep need and sleepiness at the wheel: comparative study on

French highways between 1996 and 2011. BMJ Open 2016;6(12):e012382.

22. Shekari Soleimanloo S, White MJ, Garcia-Hansen V, et al. The effects of sleep loss on young drivers' performance: a systematic review. PLoS One 2017; 12(8):e0184002.

23. Vaz Fragoso CA, Araujo KLB, Van Ness PH, et al. Sleep disturbances and adverse driving events in a predominantly male cohort of active older drivers. J Am Geriatr Soc 2010;58(10):1878–84.

24. Lévy P, Kohler M, McNicholas WT, et al. Obstructive sleep apnoea syndrome. Nat Rev Dis Primers 2015; 1:1–20.

25. Gupta R, Pandi-Perumal SR, Almeneessier AS, et al. Hypersomnolence and traffic safety. Sleep Med Clin 2017;12(3):489–99.

26. McNicholas WT, Rodenstein D. Sleep apnoea and driving risk: the need for regulation. Eur Respir Rev 2015;24(138):602–6.

27. Ward KL, Hillman DR, James A, et al. Excessive daytime sleepiness increases the risk of motor vehicle crash in obstructive sleep apnea. J Clin Sleep Med 2013;9(10):1013–21.

28. Karimi M, Hedner J, Häbel H, et al. Sleep apnea-related risk of motor vehicle accidents is reduced by continuous positive airway pressure: Swedish Traffic Accident Registry data. Sleep 2015;38(3): 341–9.

29. Kiely JL, Murphy M, McNicholas WT. Subjective efficacy of nasal CPAP therapy in obstructive sleep apnoea syndrome: a prospective controlled study. Eur Respir J 1999;13(5):1086–90.

30. Tregear S, Reston J, Schoelles K, et al. Continuous positive airway pressure reduces risk of motor vehicle crash among drivers with obstructive sleep apnea: systematic review and meta-analysis. Sleep 2010;33(10):1373–80.

31. George CF. Reduction in motor vehicle collisions following treatment of sleep apnoea with nasal CPAP. Thorax 2001;56:508–12.

32. Antonopoulos CN, Sergentanis TN, Daskalopoulou SS, et al. Nasal continuous positive airway pressure (nCPAP) treatment for obstructive sleep apnea, road traffic accidents and driving simulator performance: a meta-analysis. Sleep Med Rev 2011;15(5):301–10.

33. Pien GW, Ye L, Keenan BT, et al. Changing faces of obstructive sleep apnea: treatment effects by cluster designation in the Icelandic sleep apnea cohort. Sleep 2018;41(3):zsx201.

34. Garbarino S, Durando P, Guglielmi O, et al. Sleep apnea, sleep debt and daytime sleepiness are independently associated with road accidents. A cross-sectional study on truck drivers. PLoS One 2016; 11(11):e0166262.

35. Garbarino S, Magnavita N, Guglielmi O, et al. Insomnia is associated with road accidents. Further evidence from a study on truck drivers. PLoS One 2017;12(10):e0187256.

36. Terán-Santos J, Jimenez-Gomez A, Cordero-Guevara J. The association between sleep apnea and the risk of traffic accidents. N Engl J Med 1999;340(11):847–51.

37. Vakulin A, Baulk SD, Catcheside PG, et al. Effects of moderate sleep deprivation and low-dose alcohol on driving simulator performance and perception in young men. Sleep 2007;30(10):1327–33.

38. Marshall SC, Man-Son-Hing M. Multiple chronic medical conditions and associated driving risk: a systematic review. Traffic Inj Prev 2011;12(2):142–8.

39. Johns MW. A new method for measuring daytime sleepiness: the Epworth sleepiness scale. Sleep 1991;14(6):540–5.

40. Schreier DR, Banks C, Mathis J. Driving simulators in the clinical assessment of fitness to drive in sleepy individuals: a systematic review. Sleep Med Rev 2018;38:86–100.

41. Deegan PC, McNicholas WT. Predictive value of clinical features for the obstructive sleep apnoea syndrome. Eur Respir J 1996;9(1):117–24.

42. Kingshott RN, Sime PJ, Engleman HM, et al. Self assessment of daytime sleepiness: patient versus partner. Thorax 1995;50(9):994–5.

43. McNicholas WT, Bencs Z, De Valck E, et al. New standards and guidelines for drivers with obstructive sleep apnoea. 2013. Available at: https://ec.europa.eu/transport/road_safety/topics/behaviour/fitness_to_drive_en. Accessed September 7, 2019.

44. Kirkendoll KD, Heaton K. A policy analysis of mandatory obstructive sleep apnea screening in the trucking industry. Workplace Health Saf 2018; 66(7):348–55.

45. Burks SV, Anderson JE, Bombyk M, et al. Nonadherence with employer-mandated sleep apnea treatment and increased risk of serious truck crashes. Sleep 2016;39(5):967–75.

46. Rodenstein D, On Behalf of Cost-B26 Action on Sleep Apnoea Syndrome. Driving in Europe: the need of a common policy for drivers with obstructive sleep apnoea syndrome. J Sleep Res 2008;17(3): 281–4.

47. Revision to Annex III of EU Driving Licence Directive regarding obstructive sleep apnoea syndrome. 2014. Available at: https://eur-lex.europa.eu/legal-content/EN/TXT/?qid=1568213748387&uri=CELEX: 32014L0085. Accessed September 11, 2019.

48. Filomeno R, Ikeda A, Tanigawa T. Developing policy regarding obstructive sleep apnea and driving among commercial drivers in the United States and Japan. Ind Health 2016;54(5):469–75.

49. Rizzo D, Libman E, Creti L, et al. Determinants of policy decisions for non-commercial drivers with OSA: an integrative review. Sleep Med Rev 2018; 37:130–7.

50. Liu S-Y, Lau N, Perez MA. The impact of sleep disorders on driving safety—findings from the Second Strategic Highway Research Program naturalistic driving study. Sleep 2018;41(4). https://doi.org/10.1093/sleep/zsy023.

51. Dwarakanath A, Twiddy M, Ghosh D, et al. Variability in clinicians' opinions regarding fitness to drive in patients with obstructive sleep apnoea syndrome (OSAS). Thorax 2015;70(5):495–7.

52. Berger M, Varvarigou V, Rielly A, et al. Employer-mandated sleep apnea screening and diagnosis in commercial drivers. J Occup Environ Med 2012; 54(8):1017–25.

53. Parks PD, Durand G, Tsismenakis AJ, et al. Screening for obstructive sleep apnea during commercial driver medical examinations. J Occup Environ Med 2009;51(3):275–82.

54. Tzischinsky O, Cohen A, Doveh E, et al. Screening for sleep disordered breathing among applicants for a professional driver's license. J Occup Environ Med 2012;54(10):1275–80.

55. Zhang C, Varvarigou V, Parks PD, et al. Psychomotor vigilance testing of professional drivers in the occupational health clinic: a potential objective screen for daytime sleepiness. J Occup Environ Med 2012; 54(3):296–302.

56. Grote L, Svedmyr S, Hedner J. Certification of fitness to drive in sleep apnea patients: are we doing the right thing? J Sleep Res 2018;27(6):e12719.

57. McNicholas WT. Identifying and treating obstructive sleep apnea in sleepy drivers: everybody wins. J Sleep Res 2018;27(6):e12787.

Sleep and Transportation Safety: Role of the Employer

David Rainey, MD, MPH, MEd[a,b], Michael A. Parenteau, MD, JD, FCLM[c],
Stefanos N. Kales, MD, MPH[a,d],*

KEYWORDS

- Sleep • Fatigue • Sleep disorders • Obstructive sleep apnea • Transportation • Work • Employer

KEY POINTS

- Fatigue is a major cause of transportation accidents.
- Employers share responsibility for fatigue-related accidents, and may be legally liable for accident consequences.
- Employers play a significant role in mitigating fatigue-related risk, and may benefit by optimizing fatigue risk management.
- Multiple complementary strategies should be used for reducing fatigue-related safety risks.

INTRODUCTION

Transportation accidents remain a major cause of preventable injury and death. In 2017, transportation incidents accounted for 47% of the 5147 fatal work injuries in the United States (**Fig. 1**).[1] It was the most lethal year for heavy and tractor-trailer truck drivers since fatality data began to be recorded by occupation in 2003. Those most at risk in the transportation industry continue to be driver/sales workers and tractor-trailer truck drivers. The motoring public is also at risk of serious injury and death from trucking accidents.

Thus, the impact of fatigue and sleep disorders on transportation safety is significant. In 2014, drowsy driving was the documented cause of 82,000 crashes, 37,000 injuries, and 886 deaths (2.5% of all fatal crashes).[2] These are just the recorded numbers. The National Transportation Safety Board (NTSB) estimates drowsy driving causes 7% of all crashes and 16.5% of all fatal crashes (~5000 deaths per year).[2] Investigations by the NTSB into all transportation modes have identified that 20% of serious transportation accidents are fatigue related.[3]

A recent survey of US highway drivers found nearly half admit to falling asleep or nodding off while driving at some point during their lifetimes, and 4% report doing so in the previous 30 days.[4] Although these are sobering statistics, it is likely that the impact of sleepiness and fatigue on transportation safety is considerably higher than is currently estimated[5] because of the limitations of data collection. It is important for employers to acknowledge that professional drivers are not immune to this danger because a large proportion of all large truck crashes are estimated to be caused by drowsy or fatigued drivers.[6]

Disclosure: Dr S.N. Kales has served as a medicolegal consultant and expert witness on cases involving commercial drivers. The other authors have nothing to disclose.
[a] Occupational Medicine Residency, Harvard Medical School, Harvard TH Chan School of Public Health, Boston, MA, USA; [b] Cambridge Health Alliance Occupational Health, 5 Middlesex Avenue, Somerville, MA 02145, USA; [c] Occupational and Environmental Medicine Residency, Harvard T.H. Chan School of Public Health, 665 Huntington Avenue, Building 1, Room 1406, Boston, MA 02115, USA; [d] The Cambridge Health Alliance – Occupational Medicine, Macht Building Suite 427, 1493 Cambridge Street, Cambridge, MA 02139, USA
* Corresponding author. The Cambridge Health Alliance – Occupational Medicine, Macht Building Suite 427, 1493 Cambridge Street, Cambridge, MA 02139.
E-mail address: skales@hsph.harvard.edu

Sleep Med Clin 14 (2019) 499–508
https://doi.org/10.1016/j.jsmc.2019.08.007
1556-407X/19/© 2019 Elsevier Inc. All rights reserved.

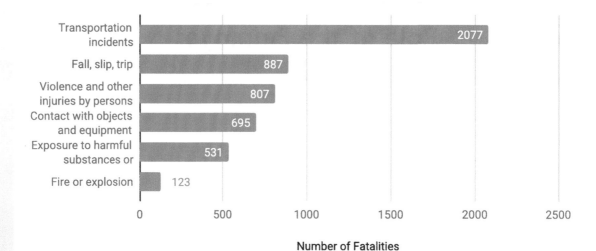

Fig. 1. Fatal occupational injuries for selected events or exposures, 2017. (*From* Bureau of Labor Statistics, Census of Fatal Occupational Injuries Summary, 2017. https://www.bls.gov/news.release/cfoi.nr0.htm.)

Employers of transportation workers have a unique opportunity and responsibility to optimize working conditions and hazard controls to prevent fatigue-related transportation accidents. They can accomplish this through a combination of sleep disorder screening and monitoring measures, engineering controls, fatigue prevention/management policies, and education.

THE EMPLOYER AS STAKEHOLDER IN FATIGUE-RELATED TRANSPORTATION SAFETY

For employers, fatigue among transportation and other safety-sensitive personnel poses a substantial risk for lost productivity, errors, and liability for damages and harm that may come to those involved in fatigue-related accidents. Such risk cannot simply be calculated as a cost of doing business, because transportation accidents can have catastrophic effects on the environment, private and public property, and loss of human life. For example, a fatigue-related operator error led to a 2010 oil tankship collision in Texas that caused $2.2 million in damages by releasing 1,749,000 L (462,000 gallons) of oil into the environment, which required evacuating 136 residents from their homes.[3,7] The NTSB determined the collision was caused by the employee's untreated obstructive sleep apnea (OSA) and work schedule. In 2015, a passenger train in New York derailed when it entered a curve where the maximum authorized speed was 30 mph (48 km/h). The train was traveling at 82 mph when it entered the curve and derailed, resulting in 4 passenger deaths and injury to more than half the remaining passengers on board. The NTSB determined that the engineer had fallen asleep because of "undiagnosed severe

OSA exacerbated by a recent circadian rhythm shift required by his work schedule."[8,9] The employer in this case was faulted for not having a medical screening policy in place for detecting sleep disorders, and for the absence of available technological controls (automated braking) to circumvent the human error.

In surveys exploring employer and employee attitudes regarding fatigue as a safety issue, employees were consistently less likely to view fatigue as a safety risk than their employers,[10] underscoring the need for increased training and awareness in the workplace around fatigue-related safety risk. Because of the frequency with which fatigue is identified as contributing to serious transportation accidents, the NTSB has issued more than 200 fatigue-related recommendations to improve transportation safety.[3] These recommendations include repeated calls for screening procedures to identify whether workers are at high risk of sleep disorders such as OSA.[9,11,12] Although no regulation currently requires screening for sleep disorders, employers would be wise to adopt such preplacement screening examinations as part of their responsibility, given they can, and have been, sued for failing to screen their workers.

These examples highlight the need for employers to recognize the crucial role they play in fatigue and sleep disorder management, as key stakeholders in transportation safety. Optimal management of sleep-related transportation safety has multiple benefits for employers. As mentioned, employers may be deemed responsible for damage caused by their employees that arise in the course of performing their jobs. When employers have appropriate measures in place to screen, treat, and eliminate fatigue-related risk, their liability is minimized, and accident rates decline significantly. In addition, companies may see financial benefits from improvements in presenteeism, health care costs, employee morale, public relations, and other less tangible rewards that support company success.

LEGAL LIABILITY OF EMPLOYERS IN TRANSPORTATION SAFETY

Employers should take a proactive approach to identify fatigued workers because they may be held legally responsible for the actions of employees if the actions resulting in injury or property damage are performed as part of their employment.[13] The legal term for this is respondeat superior, meaning "let the master answer", and this principle holds the employer vicariously liable for the acts of an employee. Vicarious liability is determined by how much the employer had the right to direct and control the employee's actions. In addition, employer liability may arise during the hiring process if employers fail to screen applicants for conditions that may impair safe operation of vehicles.[14]

Many businesses attempt to protect themselves from liability by hiring independent contractors, rather than employees. However, businesses risk losing this liability protection as they exert more control over drivers by directing the number of hours driven, routes taken, and when rest breaks are authorized.[15] At a certain point, courts will find that although the contractual relationship was characterized as an independent contract, the behaviors of the business and driver transformed it into an employer-employee relationship regardless of what was written on paper.[16]

Alternatively, when an employee works directly for the transportation employer, then the employer is usually held liable for injuries to third parties resulting from a crash.[13] This situation is especially likely when the employee has fallen asleep while operating a vehicle in the past, because it increases the foreseeability of the resulting accident.[17]

Employer policies and procedures to identify sleep disorders are critical because sleep disorders are common and employees are often unaware of their conditions.[9,14,18–20] At a minimum, it is recommended that employers refer employees with suspected sleep disorders to medical providers for assessment and treatment. OSA is the most common cause of excessive daytime sleepiness and is estimated to affect 22 million Americans, with 80% moderate to severe, but undiagnosed.[20] Screening for OSA in transportation

workers can be readily performed using objective anthropometric and medical criteria that are routinely collected as part of medical certification and preplacement medical examinations. Employers are also recommended to document having advised the worker of the increased risk of performing work-related duties while drowsy, along with potential civil or criminal responsibility, and any company policies or procedures they are expected to follow if an employee is identified as, or personally feels, too fatigued to work.

In addition to injured third parties suing the employer under a theory of vicarious liability, injured workers coming off long work days who have been injured driving home have also sued their employers.[13] Thus far, courts have not been willing to hold employers liable for worker injuries after work because the employers scheduled the worker for excessive work time.[21,22] However, given the cost of litigation, employers may want to mitigate this risk by coordinating or providing employees with transportation home at the end of long or extended shifts.

The Legal Landscape for Sleepy Drivers

In the United States there is no federal requirement to objectively screen for sleep disorders in commercial motor vehicle drivers, rail workers, or pilots. The medical examinations required for each profession typically ask a screening question such as, "Do you have sleep disorders, pauses in breathing while asleep, daytime sleepiness, loud snoring?" However, this subjective questionnaire approach has been documented as failing to capture most commercial drivers with sleep disorders because they often fail to report these symptoms even when they are present.[23,24]

If a sleep disorder is not captured on a preplacement or routine medical assessment and an accident happens, courts have generally found both the driver and the employer responsible for the accident, reasoning that sleepiness is recognizable by drivers and that accidents resulting from falling asleep are reasonably foreseeable.[25] Although most driving case law has addressed cases involving the general public and found the driver has a duty to pull off the road to rest when fatigued,[13,25] courts surely extend this expectation to commercial drivers, whom they hold to a higher standard.

An illustrative example of an employer being found liable for a sleep-related accident by one of its employees is Dunlap v W.L. Logan Trucking Co., in which the driver of a tractor trailer fell asleep at the wheel, killing a woman.[17] In this case, the court found the employee directly liable and the employer vicariously liable for the death because the employee was acting within the scope of his employment.

A more recent example occurred 2013 when a Greyhound bus went off the road in Ohio and flipped over less than an hour into its journey.[26] Six passengers were ultimately awarded $6 million for their injuries, which included compound fractures, multiple surgeries, as well as neck and back injuries. From an employer's perspective, this case is significant because the driver was evaluated for a Department of Transportation Medical Certification examination 6 weeks before the accident occurred. The examining physician determined the driver was at risk of OSA and recommended that he undergo an in-laboratory sleep study and only issued a 3-month medical certification, rather than the typical 1-year to 2-year certification that the driver had received after prior examinations. Instead of requiring the recommended sleep study, which the employer's written policy also required, the driver was directed to follow up in a medical clinic, where he was cleared of sleep apnea based only on a limited physical examination and was allowed to return to work by his employer without the requisite sleep study. Two days later, the fatigue-related accident occurred. At deposition, Greyhound's medical director acknowledged that "A physical exam alone is not going to say one way or the other whether a person has sleep apnea."[26]

For an employer invested in fatigue risk management, the identification of a driver at high risk for OSA during his medical certification should have triggered further medical review by the company's medical director, leading to compliance with the recommended diagnostic tests and possible suspension of safety-sensitive operations by that employee until they were sufficiently evaluated and treated.

Depending on where a transportation company operates, it is also important for employers to recognize that some states go beyond allowing injured parties to sue for monetary compensation. For example, Arkansas and New Jersey have laws that explicitly make it a crime to drive while drowsy, meaning the driver can go to prison for up to 10 years and face a fine up to $100,000 for vehicular homicide.[27,28] Although both of these laws require the driver to have been awake (not necessarily driving) for the preceding 24 hours for the law to apply, states such as Maine, New York, and Tennessee have all considered laws that would make it a crime if the driver is simply impaired by fatigue.[29–31] Even in places where there is no threshold established in legislation, in any tragic accident drivers may still find themselves facing a prosecutor and jury trying to decide how tired is too tired to drive. Because studies have shown people are poor judges of their own impairment from fatigue and sleepiness, it is critical that employer controls and programs are in place to identify, monitor, and manage fatigue-related safety risks.[14,18–20]

BENEFITS TO EMPLOYERS TAKING AN ACTIVE ROLE IN REDUCING FATIGUE RISK

When employers transition from taking passive positions to active roles in the management of fatigue-related risk, not only do they diminish their legal liability but their businesses stand to benefit in multiple ways. Reduction in fatigue-related accidents results in reduced costs for damages, insurance, business disruptions, and revenue loss. However, optimizing sleep can also improve productivity, employee morale, and health care cost savings. This improvement is evident in the case of Schneider National, a transportation and logistics company that successfully implemented a sleep disorder screening and management program.

As a logistics and transportation company, Schneider relies on healthy and alert drivers, and recognizes the impact that fatigue-related incidents can have on safety and the company's bottom line. In the mid-2000s, they developed a plan to overcome many of the traditional barriers that made it challenging to ensure employees with sleep disorders such as OSA were properly identified and treated. Such barriers include:

- Identifying individuals at risk of having or developing OSA
- The high cost and inconvenience of diagnostic testing via overnight polysomnography (PSG)
- The cost, discomfort, and cumbersome nature of typical OSA treatment equipment

Recognizing these obstacles, Schneider's contracted sleep health provider developed a screening program using a simple questionnaire to categorize drivers into one of 4 levels of risk for further sleep disorder testing.[32] Those in the high-risk categories would receive PSG diagnostic testing, results of which were analyzed within 24 hours. For OSA-positive employees, treatment was initiated almost immediately thereafter with equipment specifically designed to be compatible with the truck's sleeper berth. The drivers were paired with a sleep clinician and technicians for training on their new machines, along with real-time troubleshooting. Compliance with autoPAP (autoadjusting continuous positive airway pressure) treatment was objectively monitored with electronic data collection that was regularly updated. In addition, and importantly, all expenses, from diagnostic testing to treatment equipment, were covered under the employee health care plan with no out-of-pocket cost to the driver.[10,33]

The results of the program from a safety perspective were an unequivocal success. Those in the program who were fully compliant with OSA treatment were found to have a 4-fold to 5-fold lower preventable crash risk compared with comparable drivers with OSA who were never compliant with treatment, after matching for experience and miles driven. In addition, the crash rates for OSA treatment–compliant drivers were statistically no different from drivers at low risk for OSA.[33]

For Schneider, the program has also paid dividends in reducing employee turnover and improving the health of their workforce, reportedly resulting in health care plan savings of $300 to $400 per driver per month for drivers with OSA receiving treatment under the program.[10]

STEPS EMPLOYERS CAN TAKE TO MINIMIZE FATIGUE-RELATED RISK

The NTSB has issued more than 200 fatigue-related recommendations to improve transportation safety. A review by Marcus and Rosekind[3] published in 2017 categorized these recommendations into 7 focus areas:

1. Scheduling policies and practices: hours of service, time off between work assignments, company scheduling practices, and circadian disruptions.
2. Education/raising awareness: programs to increase knowledge related to human fatigue, sleep and circadian rhythms, and actions to counteract the effects of fatigue.
3. Organizational strategies: organizational activities to reduce and manage fatigue among employees, such as nonpunitive programs for employees to self-report as fatigued, or to decline work assignments because of fatigue.
4. Healthy sleep: medical issues associated with sleep disorders, such as the diagnosis and treatment of sleep apnea, or the appropriate use of medications for the treatment of insomnia.
5. Vehicle and environmental strategies: technology to detect and address operator fatigue (eg, alertness for rail crew), including adequate rest areas for commercial truck drivers.
6. Fatigue management plans: development, use, and evaluation of fatigue management plans to

manage the effects of fatigue in transportation operations.
7. Research and evaluation: topics in need of research or analysis to understand and effectively address fatigue in transportation operations.

Employers can minimize fatigue-related safety risk by addressing these focus areas.

Scheduling Policies and Practices

Approximately 30 million adults in the United States are shift workers: those who work outside the traditional 9 AM to 5 PM work day. Of these shift workers, 10% meet criteria for a shift work disorder by experiencing insomnia or excessive sleepiness during wakefulness accompanied by a reduction of total sleep time not caused by voluntary sleep restriction.[34]

Transportation workers are over-represented among shift workers, which challenges them to work safely because their natural circadian cycles diminish alertness during the performance of safety-critical tasks at night.[34] Accidents in the transportation industry also commonly result from decreased vigilance caused by excessive daytime sleepiness as a consequence of disruptions in the natural sleep-wakefulness cycles of shift workers. In addition, shiftwork and OSA cause synergistic and significant impairment.[23] Therefore, employees with OSA should preferably work during daytime hours on nonrotating shifts even when treated with CPAP.

If shiftwork is unavoidable, schedules should be informed by the latest sleep research, designed to optimize short-term and long-term health benefits and minimize sleep disturbance. For example, many chronobiologists recommend fast-forward rotating shifts, in which workers transition clockwise from day to evening to night over intervals of 2 to 3 days, with 2 to 3 days off for recovery following the night shift. The fast rotation prevents permanent shifts in circadian cycles and helps to minimize accumulation of sleep debt.[35]

Education and Training

A 2016 survey of transportation workers and their employers found that workers were less likely than their employers to consider fatigue and sleepiness to be significant safety risks.[10] Employers can help raise awareness of fatigue as a major factor in transportation safety and the measures they are taking to mitigate the risk. Sleep hygiene and fatigue management training should be incorporated into safety training and monitoring programs. In addition, employers can educate workers on the health benefits the employees can reap as individuals by making healthy sleep an integral part of their personal and professional responsibilities.

Organizational Strategies

Employers should create a culture in which fatigue-related safety is valued and supported by policies and practices. Care must be taken so as not to create perverse incentives, whereby employees may be penalized for not continuing to work when too fatigued or sleepy to do so. For example, members of the Owner-Operator Independent Drivers Association have expressed concern that regulations designed to keep them safe can paradoxically force them to stay on the road when dispatchers at companies that hire their services cite these regulations in support of assigning additional tasks, without regard to road and traffic conditions, weather, and driver fatigue that may jeopardize safety.[36] These drivers express feeling compelled to accept these assignments despite fatigue or adverse conditions, because the employer expects they can work to the limits of the regulation. Employers should keep in mind that although the Federal Motor Carrier Safety Administration (FMCSA) regulations were established to limit sleepy drivers on the road, complying with the regulations does not guarantee a driver will not be fatigued, and employers are encouraged to trust their drivers when they are tired or in adverse road conditions.

Healthy Sleep: Identifying and Treating Sleep Disorders

Employers should screen individuals considered for safety-sensitive positions for sleep disorders, including OSA. Employers should be concerned about untreated OSA because it has been linked to $65 billion to $165 billion in costs caused by lost productivity as well as increased health and safety costs and higher rates of accidents.[6]

Objective screening criteria are preferred because commercial drivers usually do not report their symptoms because of concerns (perceived or real) of the negative economic and occupational impact of an OSA diagnosis.[6,23] These concerns range from the inconvenience of diagnostic testing and treatment to loss of income and employment. Accordingly, screening should use and rely primarily on objective risk factors such as male gender, age, body mass index (BMI), neck circumference, and hypertension, rather than subjective self-reported symptoms.

Although not required by regulation,[11] to mitigate the significant threat of substantial harm to employees and the general public, employers should

require safety-sensitive transit workers to undergo testing for OSA who meet the following criteria[37]:

- All people with BMI ≥40
- All people with a BMI 33 to 40 and 3 or more of the following:
  - Male or postmenopausal female
  - Age ≥42 years
  - Neck circumference
    - Greater than 43 cm (17 inches) for men
    - Greater than 39.5 cm (15.5 inches) for women
  - Mallampati class 3 or 4
  - Witnessed apneas
  - Loud snoring
  - Micrognathia or retrognathia
  - Hypertension (treated or untreated)
  - Type 2 diabetes (treated or untreated)
  - Hypothyroidism (untreated)
  - History of stroke, coronary artery disease, or arrhythmia

Workers diagnosed with OSA should be disqualified from safety-sensitive tasks until they are successfully treated.

Employers in the transportation industry and their occupational physicians should be vigilant regarding the medications their workers are taking because many can affect daytime alertness. As a general rule, medications depressing the central nervous system deserve careful deliberation in transportation workers because they can adversely affect safety-sensitive duties.[34] In addition, although there may be temptation to prescribe wake-promoting stimulants (eg, modafinil, armodafinil), these are not a substitute for fatigue prevention and management strategies, and should only be used in specific cases with expert guidance as adjuncts.

FMCSA regulation section 391.41(b)(12) states:

A person is physically qualified to drive a commercial motor vehicle (CMV) if that person does not use a controlled substance identified in 21 CFR 1308.11, Schedule I, an amphetamine, a narcotic, or any other habit-forming drug. Exception: A driver may use such a substance or drug, if the substance or drug is prescribed by a licensed medical practitioner who is familiar with the driver's medical history and assigned duties; and has advised the driver that the prescribed substance or drug will not adversely affect the driver's ability to safely operate a CMV. This exception does not apply to methadone.

Medical examiners are required to carefully assess the effects of a driver's medications on their ability to operate a vehicle safely before qualifying the driver to do so commercially.

Employee education is also critical in this regard, because common over-the-counter medications, supplements, and legally obtained prescriptions may be disqualifying when they adversely affect the driver's ability to drive safely.[38–45]

Table 1 gives guidance to prescribing physicians providing care to transportation workers regarding common medications that have sedating side effects,[34] which the FMCSA advises against in transportation workers, and offers alternatives that could be considered.

Technology/Engineering Controls

As with any hazard, if elimination of risk is not possible, engineering controls to mitigate risk are desirable rather than relying on individual human factors or performance, such as the application of personal protective equipment or safety practices (eg, the strategic use of caffeine and napping) to effectively minimize the hazard. Employers in the transportation industry can use increasingly sophisticated systems to detect and even compensate for sleepy drivers and operators. For example, an automated braking system at rail stations and turns acts as an operator-independent failsafe against speed-related derailments or crashes, which have caused catastrophic accidents in the past. As automated driving technologies mature in the coming years, employers in the trucking industry can integrate technologies that both detect driver fatigue and intervene to keep them alert, and also take control of the vehicle to avoid lane departures, speeding, and

Table 1
Common sedating medications and potential alternatives

Sedating Medication	Alternative
First-generation antihistamines (eg, diphenhydramine)	Second-generation antihistamines (eg, loratadine and cetirizine)[39]
Sedating antidepressants (eg, mirtazapine, trazodone, imipramine, amitriptyline)	Nonsedating antidepressants (eg, sertraline, citalopram,[40] venlafaxine, bupropion)[39]
Narcotic pain medications (eg, opiates/opioids). Many are explicitly banned for commercial drivers (eg, methadone)[39]	Pain medications (eg, acetaminophen,[41] NSAIDs,[42] COX-2 inhibitors)
Hypnotics (eg, benzodiazepines, barbiturates)	Do not drive until drug is cleared from the body (ie, after 7 half-lives for acute use and 7 half-lives + 1 wk for chronic use). Sleep aid (melatonin: do not drive within 8 h of taking)[43]
Anxiolytics (eg, diazepam, lorazepam)	In general, not recommended by FMCSA
Muscle relaxants (eg, cyclobenzaprine)	In general, not recommended within 6 d of driving
Sedating anticonvulsants (eg, gabapentin, carbamazepine)	In general, use of these medications precludes medical certification if prescribed for epilepsy or other disqualifying conditions outlined by the FMCSA
Antipsychotics (eg, quetiapine, risperidone, olanzapine)	In general, use of these medications precludes medical certification if prescribed for disqualifying conditions outlined by the FMCSA If the underlying condition being treated is safe for driving and medication use for the driver is effective, safe, and stable, clearance may be considered for less sedating atypical antipsychotics (eg, risperidone, olanzapine, quetiapine, and ziprasidone)[44]
Dopamine agonists for Parkinson disease (eg, pramipexole, ropinirole, pergolide)	In general, not recommended because they may cause narcolepsylike attacks
Marijuana, prescribed medically (remains federally banned)	Does not qualify for FMCSA medical certification[45]

Abbreviations: COX-2, cyclooxygenase-2; NSAIDs, nonsteroidal antiinflammatory drugs.

collisions. This technology is increasingly available in consumer vehicles, and can assist with lane control, warning when an obstacle is ahead, and braking before a collision is detected by the driver. Other available technologies include computer-analyzed steering wheel movements to detect when a driver is fatigued, but before the driver falls asleep. Devices that directly monitor a driver's eyes or electrodermal activity can also detect fatigue before the driver falls asleep, triggering an alert to arouse the driver. It is anticipated that such technological engineering controls will play an integral role in improving transportation safety in the future.

Fatigue Management Plans

Fatigue management plans organize and formalize employers' efforts to minimize fatigue-related risk. They should include statements of intent and scope; clearly delineate work hours and overtime policies; identify fatigue-related safety issues; and outline mitigation strategies, including training, medical screening, engineering controls, and strategies for reporting and investigating fatigue-related incidents and near misses.

For fatigue management plans to succeed, they must be science based, data driven for the specific transit industry, cooperatively designed by all stakeholders, integrated into a culture of workplace safety and health management, and continuously improved using feedback and evaluation.[46] Senior leadership must nurture a culture of trust between managers and workers as well as having accountability for the program.[6] A successful program will not only improve fatigue-related safety risk but also improve morale, productivity, work satisfaction, and well-being for employees and for the company.

Research and Evaluation

In addition, as in all endeavors, ongoing research is integral to deepening the understanding of fatigue-related safety risk; its impact on employers, workers, and the public; and what methods are optimal for its mitigation. As shown by Schneider National, private corporations can collaborate in numerous ways with the scientific research community to further the collective understanding of how fatigue-related risk can be minimized in transportation safety. Employers of all sizes can contribute to ongoing research in numerous ways, including data collection, active collaborations with researchers, and through financial support of ongoing research. At a minimum, employers should analyze their own safety data, regularly evaluate their fatigue management plans, collect feedback from stakeholders, and track progress.

SUMMARY

Despite tremendous progress that has been made in transportation safety over the past century, transportation incidents remain one of the leading causes of industrial accidents, often with serious adverse consequences to human life, public property, and the environment. Human fatigue is increasingly recognized as an important factor in transportation safety, and employers play a vital role with their employees in ensuring fatigue-related risk is minimized. The NTSB has identified 7 focus areas employers can address to reduce fatigue-related transportation safety risk. By taking an active role as stakeholders in transportation safety, employers not only reduce their risk of adverse safety events and limit their legal liability but may also benefit from improvements in productivity, morale, and health care costs, all of which contribute to a healthier workforce, healthier companies, and safer travel for everyone.

REFERENCES

1. Bureau of Labor Statistics, Census of fatal occupational injuries summary, 2017. Available at: https://www.bls.gov/news.release/cfoi.nr0.htm. Accessed January 27, 2019.
2. Research on Drowsy Driving | National Highway Traffic Safety Administration (NHTSA). Available at: https://one.nhtsa.gov/Driving-Safety/Drowsy-Driving/Research-on-Drowsy-Driving. Accessed February 18, 2019.
3. Marcus JH, Rosekind MR. Fatigue in transportation: NTSB investigations and safety recommendations. Inj Prev 2017;23(4):232–8.
4. Prevalence of motor vehicle crashes involving drowsy drivers, United States, 2009-2013. AAA Foundation; 2014. Available at: https://aaafoundation.org/prevalence-motor-vehicle-crashes-involving-drowsy-drivers-united-states-2009-2013/. Accessed January 26, 2019.
5. Currin A. Drowsy driving. NHTSA 2016. Available at: https://www.nhtsa.gov/risky-driving/drowsy-driving. Accessed January 27, 2019.
6. Zhang C, Berger MB, Rielly A, et al. Chapter 79 - obstructive sleep apnea in the workplace. In: Kryger M, Roth T, Dement WC, editors. Principles and practice of sleep medicine. 6th edition. Philadelphia: Elsevier; 2017. p. 750–6.e4. https://doi.org/10.1016/B978-0-323-24288-2.00079-9.
7. Collision of tankship eagle otome with cargo vessel gull arrow and subsequent collision with the dixie vengeance tow sabine-neches canal, Port Arthur,

Texas. 2010. Available at: https://www.ntsb.gov/investigations/AccidentReports/Reports/MAR1104.pdf. Accessed January 27, 2019.

8. Railroad accident brief RAB1412. Available at: https://www.ntsb.gov/investigations/AccidentReports/Pages/RAB1412.aspx. Accessed January 27, 2019.

9. NYC commuter railroad crashes spur NTSB to renew call for sleep apnea screenings. 2018. Available at: https://www.safetyandhealthmagazine.com/articles/16661-nyc-commuter-railroad-crashes-spur-ntsb-to-renew-call-for-sleep-apnea-screenings. Accessed January 27, 2019.

10. Council NS. Fatigue report (Part 3) - in safety-critical industries | National Safety Council. Available at: http://safety.nsc.org/fatigue-in-safety-critical-industries-report. Accessed January 24, 2019.

11. Colvin LJ, Collop NA. Commercial motor vehicle driver obstructive sleep apnea screening and treatment in the United States: an update and recommendation overview. J Clin Sleep Med 2016;12(1):113–25.

12. Kales SN, Czeisler CA. Obstructive sleep apnea and work accidents: time for action. Sleep 2016;39(6):1171–3.

13. Brown D. Legal obligations of persons who have sleep disorders or who treat or hire them. In: Kryger M, Roth T, Dement WC, editors. Principles and practice of sleep medicine. 6th edition. Philadelphia: Elsevier; 2016. p. 661–6.

14. Venkateshiah S, Hoque R, DelRosso L. Legal and regulatory aspects of sleep disorders. Sleep Med Clin 2017;12(1):149–60.

15. In re Van Dusen, 654 F.3d 838 (9th Cir. 2011).

16. New Prime, Inc. v. Oliveira, 138 S.Ct. 1164 (2018).

17. Dunlap v. W.L. Logan Trucking Co. 2005.

18. United States. Department Of Transportation. Bureau Of Transportation Statistics. Transportation Statistics Annual Report 2018. Available. 2018. https://doi.org/10.21949/1502596.

19. Carden K, Malhotra A. The debate about gender differences in obstructive sleep apnea. Sleep Med 2003;4(6):485–7.

20. Institute of Medicine (US) Committee on Sleep Medicine and Research. In: Colten HR, Altevogt BM, editors. Sleep disorders and sleep deprivation: an unmet public health problem. Washington, DC: National Academies Press (US); 2006. Available at: http://www.ncbi.nlm.nih.gov/books/NBK19960/. Accessed January 25, 2019.

21. Black v. William Insulation Co. 2006.

22. Barclay v. Briscoe, 47 A.3d 560, 427 Md. 270; (Md., 2012).

23. Kales SN, Straubel MG. Obstructive sleep apnea in North American commercial drivers. Ind Health 2014;52(1):13–24.

24. Johns MW. A new method for measuring daytime sleepiness: the Epworth sleepiness scale. Sleep 1991;14(6):540–5.

25. Bushnell v. Bushnell, 103 CONN. 583, 131 A. 432 (1925).

26. Ruthie Alle. v. Greyhound Lines, Inc.(Co. Ct. at Law No. 3, Dallas County, Texas 2015). Available at: http://files.courthousenews.com/2016/03/09/Greyhound%20Sleep.pdf).

27. N.J.S.A. x 2C:11–5(a).

28. ARKANSAS CODE x 5-10-105.

29. Maine: HB 683 (2015).

30. New York: AB 692 (2015).

31. Tennessee: SB 2586 (2014).

32. Berger M, Varvarigou V, Rielly A, et al. Employer-mandated sleep apnea screening and diagnosis in commercial drivers. J Occup Environ Med 2012;54(8):1017–25.

33. Burks SV, Anderson JE, Bombyk M, et al. Nonadherence with employer-mandated sleep apnea treatment and increased risk of serious truck crashes. Sleep 2016;39(5):967–75.

34. Cheng P, Drake C. Occupational sleep medicine. Sleep Med Clin 2016;11(1):65–79.

35. Burgess PA. Optimal shift duration and sequence: recommended approach for short-term emergency response activations for public health and emergency management. Am J Public Health 2007;97(Suppl 1):S88–92.

36. OOIDA press release, owner-operator independent drivers association. Owner Operator Independent Drivers Association, Trucking Association. Available at: https://www.ooida.com/MediaCenter/Press Releases/pressrelease.asp. Accessed January 18, 2019.

37. Proposed recommendations on obstructive sleep apnea. Federal Register. 2012. Available at: https://www.federalregister.gov/documents/2012/04/20/2012-9555/proposed-recommendations-on-obstructive-sleep-apnea. Accessed February 18, 2019.

38. Can a CMV driver be disqualified for using a legally prescribed drug? Federal Motor Carrier Safety Administration. 2014. Available at: https://www.fmcsa.dot.gov/faq/can-cmv-driver-be-disqualified-using-legally-prescribed-drug. Accessed January 18, 2019.

39. FMCSA Medical Examiner Handbook. 260.

40. Hansen S. Antidepressant choices in primary care: which to use first? Wis Med J 2004;103(6):93–8.

41. Nagai J, Uesawa Y, Shimamura R, et al. Characterization of the adverse effects induced by acetaminophen and nonsteroidal anti-inflammatory drugs based on the analysis of the Japanese adverse drug event report database. Clin J Pain 2017;33(8):667–75.

42. Sostres C, Gargallo CJ, Arroyo MT, et al. Adverse effects of non-steroidal anti-inflammatory drugs (NSAIDs, aspirin and coxibs) on upper gastrointestinal tract. Best Pract Res Clin Gastroenterol 2010;24(2):121–32.

43. Suhner A, Schlagenhauf P, Tschopp A, et al. Impact of melatonin on driving performance. J Travel Med 1998;5(1):7–13.

44. Miller DD. Atypical antipsychotics: sleep, sedation, and efficacy. Prim Care Companion J Clin Psychiatry 2004;6(Suppl 2):3–7.

45. Can a driver meet the qualification standards under 49 CFR § 391.41(b)(12) if using medical marijuana. Federal Motor Carrier Safety Administration. 2017. Available at: https://www.fmcsa.dot.gov/faq/can-driver-meet-qualification-standards-under-49-cfr-%C2%A7-39141b12-if-using-medical-marijuan. Accessed January 18, 2019.

46. Lerman SE, Eskin E, Flower DJ, et al. Fatigue risk management in the workplace. J Occup Environ Med 2012;54(2):231–58.

UNITED STATES POSTAL SERVICE®
Statement of Ownership, Management, and Circulation (All Periodicals Publications Except Requester Publications)

1. Publication Title: SLEEP MEDICINE CLINICS

2. Publication Number: 025 – 053

3. Filing Date: 9/18/2019

4. Issue Frequency: MAR, JUN, SEP, DEC

5. Number of Issues Published Annually: 4

6. Annual Subscription Price: $212.00

7. Complete Mailing Address of Known Office of Publication (Not printer) (Street, city, county, state, and ZIP+4®)
ELSEVIER INC.
230 Park Avenue, Suite 800
New York, NY 10169

Contact Person: STEPHEN R. BUSHING
Telephone (Include area code): 215-239-3688

8. Complete Mailing Address of Headquarters or General Business Office of Publisher (Not printer)
ELSEVIER INC.
230 Park Avenue, Suite 800
New York, NY 10169

9. Full Names and Complete Mailing Addresses of Publisher, Editor, and Managing Editor (Do not leave blank)

Publisher (Name and complete mailing address)
TAYLOR BALL, ELSEVIER INC.
1600 JOHN F KENNEDY BLVD. SUITE 1800
PHILADELPHIA, PA 19103-2899

Editor (Name and complete mailing address)
COLLEEN DIETZLER, ELSEVIER INC.
1600 JOHN F KENNEDY BLVD. SUITE 1800
PHILADELPHIA, PA 19103-2899

Managing Editor (Name and complete mailing address)
PATRICK MANLEY, ELSEVIER INC.
1600 JOHN F KENNEDY BLVD. SUITE 1800
PHILADELPHIA, PA 19103-2899

10. Owner (Do not leave blank. If the publication is owned by a corporation, give the name and address of the corporation immediately followed by the names and addresses of all stockholders owning or holding 1 percent or more of the total amount of stock. If not owned by a corporation, give the names and addresses of the individual owners. If owned by a partnership or other unincorporated firm, give its name and address as well as those of each individual owner. If the publication is published by a nonprofit organization, give its name and address.)

Full Name	Complete Mailing Address
WHOLLY OWNED SUBSIDIARY OF REED/ELSEVIER, US HOLDINGS	1600 JOHN F KENNEDY BLVD. SUITE 1800 PHILADELPHIA, PA 19103-2899

11. Known Bondholders, Mortgagees, and Other Security Holders Owning or Holding 1 Percent or More of Total Amount of Bonds, Mortgages, or Other Securities. If none, check box ► ☐ None

Full Name	Complete Mailing Address
N/A	

12. Tax Status (For completion by nonprofit organizations authorized to mail at nonprofit rates) (Check one)
The purpose, function, and nonprofit status of this organization and the exempt status for federal income tax purposes:
☒ Has Not Changed During Preceding 12 Months
☐ Has Changed During Preceding 12 Months (Publisher must submit explanation of change with this statement)

PS Form **3526**, July 2014 [Page 1 of 4 (see instructions page 4)] PSN: 7530-01-000-9931 PRIVACY NOTICE: See our privacy policy on www.usps.com.

---

13. Publication Title: SLEEP MEDICINE CLINICS

14. Issue Date for Circulation Data Below: JUNE 2019

15. Extent and Nature of Circulation

		Average No. Copies Each Issue During Preceding 12 Months	No. Copies of Single Issue Published Nearest to Filing Date
a. Total Number of Copies (Net press run)		231	251
b. Paid Circulation (By Mail and Outside the Mail)	(1) Mailed Outside-County Paid Subscriptions Stated on PS Form 3541 (Include paid distribution above nominal rate, advertiser's proof copies, and exchange copies)	149	183
	(2) Mailed In-County Paid Subscriptions Stated on PS Form 3541 (Include paid distribution above nominal rate, advertiser's proof copies, and exchange copies)	0	0
	(3) Paid Distribution Outside the Mails Including Sales Through Dealers and Carriers, Street Vendors, Counter Sales, and Other Paid Distribution Outside USPS®	30	37
	(4) Paid Distribution by Other Classes of Mail Through the USPS (e.g. First-Class Mail®)	0	0
c. Total Paid Distribution (Sum of 15b (1), (2), (3), and (4))		179	220
d. Free or Nominal Rate Distribution (By Mail and Outside the Mail)	(1) Free or Nominal Rate Outside-County Copies Included on PS Form 3541	39	18
	(2) Free or Nominal Rate In-County Copies Included on PS Form 3541	0	0
	(3) Free or Nominal Rate Copies Mailed at Other Classes Through the USPS (e.g. First-Class Mail)	0	0
	(4) Free or Nominal Rate Distribution Outside the Mail (Carriers or other means)	0	0
e. Total Free or Nominal Rate Distribution (Sum of 15d (1), (2), (3) and (4))		39	18
f. Total Distribution (Sum of 15c and 15e)		218	238
g. Copies not Distributed (See Instructions to Publishers #4 (page #3))		13	13
h. Total (Sum of 15f and g)		231	251
i. Percent Paid (15c divided by 15f times 100)		82.11%	92.44%

* If you are claiming electronic copies, go to line 16 on page 3. If you are not claiming electronic copies, skip to line 17 on page 3.

PS Form **3526**, July 2014 (Page 2 of 4)

16. Electronic Copy Circulation

	Average No. Copies Each Issue During Preceding 12 Months	No. Copies of Single Issue Published Nearest to Filing Date
a. Paid Electronic Copies ►		
b. Total Paid Print Copies (Line 15c) + Paid Electronic Copies (Line 16a) ►		
c. Total Print Distribution (Line 15f) + Paid Electronic Copies (Line 16a) ►		
d. Percent Paid (Both Print & Electronic Copies) (16b divided by 16c × 100) ►		

☒ I certify that 50% of all my distributed copies (electronic and print) are paid above a nominal price.

17. Publication of Statement of Ownership
☒ If the publication is a general publication, publication of this statement is required. Will be printed in the DECEMBER 2019 issue of this publication. ☐ Publication not required.

18. Signature and Title of Editor, Publisher, Business Manager, or Owner

STEPHEN R. BUSHING - INVENTORY DISTRIBUTION CONTROL MANAGER

Date: 9/18/2019

I certify that all information furnished on this form is true and complete. I understand that anyone who furnishes false or misleading information on this form or who omits material or information requested on the form may be subject to criminal sanctions (including fines and imprisonment) and/or civil sanctions (including civil penalties).

PS Form **3526**, July 2014 (Page 3 of 4) PRIVACY NOTICE: See our privacy policy on www.usps.com.

Moving?

Make sure your subscription moves with you!

To notify us of your new address, find your **Clinics Account Number** (located on your mailing label above your name), and contact customer service at:

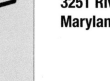

Email: journalscustomerservice-usa@elsevier.com

800-654-2452 (subscribers in the U.S. & Canada)
314-447-8871 (subscribers outside of the U.S. & Canada)

Fax number: 314-447-8029

Elsevier Health Sciences Division
Subscription Customer Service
3251 Riverport Lane
Maryland Heights, MO 63043

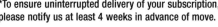

*To ensure uninterrupted delivery of your subscription, please notify us at least 4 weeks in advance of move.

ELSEVIER

Printed and bound by CPI Group (UK) Ltd, Croydon, CR0 4YY

03/10/2024

01040308-0009